LOW VISION:
ASSESSMENT AND
EDUCATIONAL NEEDS

LOW VISION: ASSESSMENT AND EDUCATIONAL NEEDS

A GUIDE TO TEACHERS AND PARENTS

DR. G. VICTORIA NAOMI

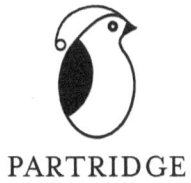

PARTRIDGE

ISBN: Softcover   978-1-4828-8968-0
               eBook   978-1-4828-8967-3

Print information available on the last page.

To order additional copies of this book, contact
Partridge India
000 800 10062 62
orders.india@partridgepublishing.com

www.partridgepublishing.com/india

Contents

CHAPTER I

Structure of eye and implications of low vision

Parts of Eye

Eye is the predominant sense organ of human being. It is a very sensitive organ in our body to be taken care of properly. Around 85 per cent of the information are received through our eyes. Sight is the sense through which the brain receives approximately 75% of its information. The eye collects information about size, shape and colour and transmits those to brain where these are interpreted. The process by which the brain interprets information received from the eye is called vision. Vision is possible only if light is present. Light rays reflected received by the eye are converted into electrical impulses and interpreted in brain. Such a precious eye is given care so as to avoid vision loss.

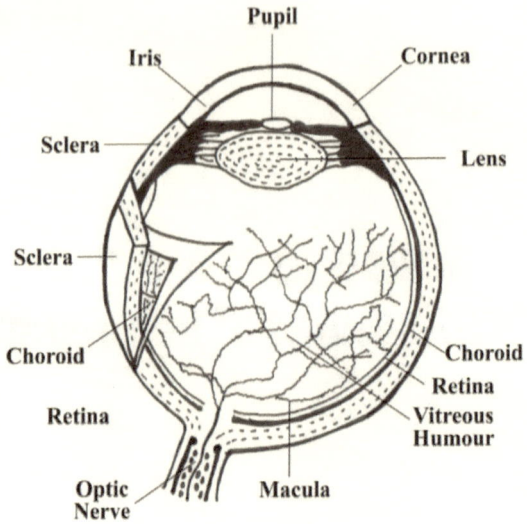

Structure of the Eye

The eyeball is 23-24 mm in length. It has three coats namely outer coat (Sclera), middle vascular coat (Uveal tract) and inner nervous coat (Retina).

Outer coat

Sclera is the outer coat of the eye. The white portion of the eye which one sees from the front is a part of Sclera. It forms 5/6th portion of the outer coat of the eye ball. The remaining 1/6th portion in front of the sclera is the Cornea. It is transparent and sits over the sclera like a watch glass. The cornea is continuous with the sclera at the sclero-corneal margin called the limbus. The anterior part of the sclera is covered by a mucous membrane called Conjunctiva which is reflected over the lids. Inner surface of the sclera is brown and lies in contact with the choroid underneath.

Middle vascular coat

It is also called as the Uveal tract. It consists of iris, ciliary body and choroid. The anterior part called iris which rests on the lens. In the centre of the iris there is a hole called pupil which regulates the entrance of light into the eye. The middle part called the ciliary body which has ciliary muscles and ciliary processes. Ciliary muscles are responsible for accommodation and cliliary processes are responsible for secreting aqueous humour. The posterior part called the choroid which lies on the inner side of sclera. The function of the choroid is to supply nutrition to the retina.

Inner nervous coat

Inner nervous coat is called Retina. It acts like the film of a camera. The retina contains millions of pigment cells. These cells are known as rods and cones which are light-receiving cells (photoreceptors). The nerve fibres arising from the eye ball converge posteriorly to form the optic nerve.

Chambers

The iris sits between the **anterior chamber** and the **posterior chamber** in the front part of the eye. These chambers contain a watery liquid known as **aqueous humour**, which is constantly being produced (by the **ciliary body**) and drained away. Aqueous humour is important for nourishing the lens and cornea.

Different Parts and Functions of the Eye

Iris
The coloured part of the eye which controls the entry of light by changing the size of the pupil.

Pupil
The 'black hole' in the centre of the iris through which light rays enter the eye.

Cornea
The clear window at the front of the eye. The cornea does most of the focusing of light rays on to the retina.

Lens
A disc-shaped structure inside the front of the eye which changes shape to focus light rays coming into the eye. Usually the lens is transparent.

Sclera
The tough, white outer coating of the eyeball.

Vitreous humour
The transparent jelly-like fluid which fills most of the volume of the eye.

Retina
The innermost layer of the eye containing cells which convert light into an electrical signal transmitted to the brain for processing into sight.

Rods

There are 125 million rod cells in the eye that are responsible for night vision and peripheral (side) vision. Disorders of the rods produce night blindness and tunnel vision.

Cones

There are about 7 million cone cells. They are concentrated in the macula and are responsible for day vision, fine central vision and colour vision. Disorders of the cones produce poor central vison, loss of colour vision and an increased sensitivity to light.

Choroid

The layer of the eye immediately behind the retina. It consists of blood vessels which nourish the outer part of the retina.

Macula

The small central part of the retina specialised for colour and fine detail vision. The centre of the macula is called the fovea.

Optic nerve

The cable of nerve fibres which carry messages from the retina to the visual centres of the brain.

Visual cortex

The part of the brain which receives electrical signals from the eyes. Vision is a function of the cerebral cortex. The eye converts light into an electrical signal (similar to the way a TV camera works). The visual cortex is where we actually see (similar to the TV station).

Visual pathways

The parts of the brain carrying visual information. The primary visual pathway extends from the eye to the mid-brain and then on to the visual cortex at the back of the brain.

Major Causes of Low Vision

Albinism

Albinism is a hereditary condition in which there is a lack of pigment in the eyes and, in some cases, in the hair and skin as well. Students with albinism are sensitive to light. Albinism is almost always associated with nystagmus. Hats and blockout sunscreen should be considered for outdoors, and parents consulted about protection against the sun.

Cataracts

Cataracts are an opacity in the lens of the eye. In cases when the normally clear lens becomes cloudy, glare can be a great problem. Students with cataracts often perform better in reduced lighting conditions. When outdoors, hats and/ or tinted glasses should be worn.

Some cataracts are surgically removed. Following successful cataract surgery, glasses or contact lenses are prescribed to restore useful vision. There are also many cases of congenital cataracts that are not severe enough to require surgery.

Optic atrophy

Atrophy in any portion of the optic nerve affects the transmission of visual impulses to the rain's visual centres. Images are hazy and indeterminate and often there is a loss of visual fields. Colour vision may also be affected. Optic atrophy has many causes including injury, infection and inherited conditions.

Macular degeneration

The macula is responsible for fine, detailed vision and colour differentiation. With this condition, deterioration of the macular area of the retina can occur suddenly, resulting in impairment of central vision.

As central vision is affected, small print often cannot be seen without low vision aids and it may be necessary to enlarge some materials. Peripheral vision which is used for mobility is usually retained.

Retinitis pigmentosa

This condition refers to a group of disorders of the retina which have the common effect of reducing peripheral vision. This results in tunnel vision and problems with night vision.

Central vision is usually retained until late in the course of the disease. Students with this condition usually read small print but may have mobility problems due to restricted visual fields.

Refractive Errors

a. **Nearsightedness**: it is also called myopia. In this condition, the person can see clearly up close but blurry in the distance.

b. **Farsightedness**: it is also called hyperopia. In this condition the person can see clearly in the distance but blurry up close.

c. **Presbyopia**: If the person is older than 40 years of age and have trouble reading small print or focusing up close, this is usually due to a condition called presbyopia.

d. **Astigmatism** is another condition that causes blurred vision, but it is because of the shape of the cornea. These conditions affect the shape of the eye and, in turn, how the eye sees. They can be corrected by eyeglasses, contact lenses, and in some cases surgery.

Crossed Eyes (strabismus)

Strabismus occurs when the eyes do not line up or they are crossed. One eye, however, usually remains straight at any given time. Common forms of strabismus include:

- Esotropia - one or both eyes turn inward toward the nose
- Exotropia - one or both eyes turn out; also called wall-eyed
- Hypertropia - one or both eyes turn up
- Hypotropia - one or both eyes turn down

If detected early in life, strabismus can be treated and even reverse. If left untreated strabismus can cause amblyopia.

Amblyopia (Lazy Eye)

Amblyopic is caused when the brain and the eye not working together. The brain ignores visual information from one eye causing problems with vision development. Treatment for amblyopia works well if the condition is found early. If treatment is done early, amblyopia leads to permanent vision loss. The risk factors for amblyopia include premature birth, low birth weight, retinopathy of prematurity diagnosis, maternal smoking, drug or alcohol use, cerebral palsy diagnosis, family history of certain eye conditions

Characteristics of Low Vision Children

Low vision is not blindness, which is the absence of useful vision. Persons with low vision may see light, color, movement, dimension, shape and size. However, things can appear blurred, faded or distorted. A person's visual acuity-the ability to see fine detail-can worsen. There can be a narrowing or loss of parts of the visual field-the area of sight. Someone with low vision may be less sensitive to differences and changes in brightness, contrast and color. Adaptation to high or low levels of light may be slowed or impossible. Various combinations of these changes in vision can occur.

Most students with low vision can use print for learning. Some may need visual aids such as glasses and other magnifying devices. Depending on the eye condition and the task, each child will have different needs. For example, one child may have sufficient vision to move around freely, but be unable to distinguish small print or facial features; another may be able to read small print but not able to see detail beyond a relatively a short distance; another may have such reduced vision that parts of objects or words are visible. Most children with low vision will have difficulty reading on the black board without the help of a low vision aid.

Some of these children may wear glasses which help improve their vision, but cannot be corrected to normal levels.

Low vision: classification

Low vision can be classified into (1) severe ability loss, (2) moderate ability loss, and (3) mild ability loss, depending on the visual function.

Moderate ability loss

Objects visible to children with normal vision at or beyond 120 metres can only be seen by children with severe low vision at 6 metres, or their visual field is 20 degrees or less.

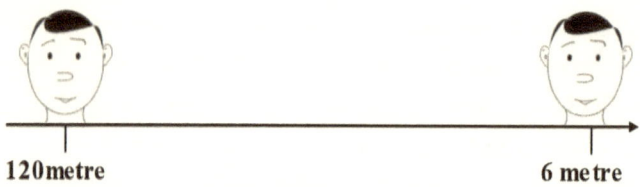

120metre   6 metre

Severe ability loss

Objects visible to children with normal vision within 60 to 120 metres can only be seen by children with moderate low vision at 6 metres.

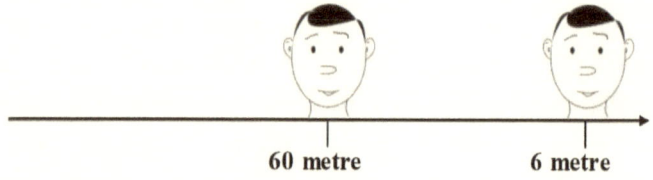

60 metre   6 metre

Mild ability loss

Objects visible to children with normal vision within 18 to 60 metres can only be seen by children with mild low vision at 6 metres.

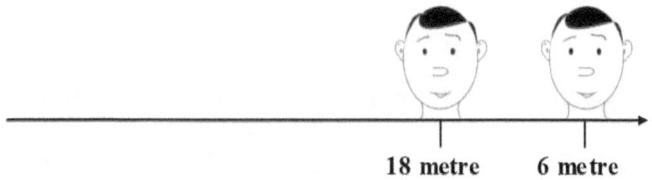

Implication of Low Vision

There are literally hundreds of different eye diseases that cause visual impairment. The first concept is to consider that every eye disease can be placed in one or more of these three categories of vision loss based on the similarity of functional symptoms. They are:

1. Blurred vision - over all blurred or hazy vision
2. Peripheral field loss - vision loss at the sides
3. Central field loss - vision loss of the central part

The following image demonstrates what type of vision loss the low vision persons experience based on the functional symptom.

Dr. G. Victoria Naomi

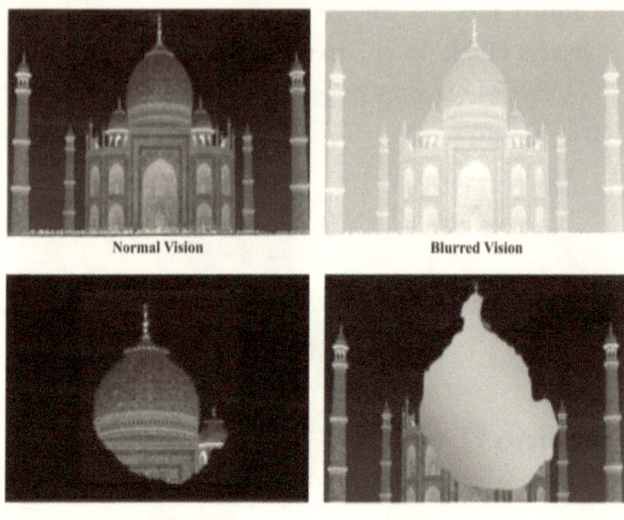

Normal Vision   Blurred Vision

Peripheral Vision Loss   Central Vision Loss

Students with low vision exhibit a wide range of visual impairments. Teachers should be aware that no two students with low vision have the same functional vision even if they are diagnosed as having the same eye condition and similar vision acuity. Vision may fluctuate and be influenced by such factors as fatigue, light glare, lighting conditions and time of day. Therefore, special attention must be given in assessing the needs of the student with low vision. Accommodations can be incorporated into his/her program plan.

Psychosocial Issues

Another issue relating to low vision is the psychosocial impact of a visual impairment. Children growing up with a visual impairment can experience many negative consequences including:

- feeling like they look different, either because they cannot visually verify how others look or because they wear glasses or use optical devices,
- feeling like an outsider because they cannot take part fully in activities,
- feeling less than capable because they do not understand visual concepts fully,
- feeling clumsy because they drop things or bump into objects.

All of these consequences can have the effect of lowering self-esteem. It is important that students identify themselves not by their visual impairment but see their visual impairment as one aspect of who they are. Intervention may be necessary so that a student can build successful experiences and find activities in which they excel.

Common Misconceptions about Vision

Glasses always help correct low vision

Some students with low vision will be helped by corrective lenses, vision will not be corrected to normal levels. There are many students with low vision who would not benefit from corrective lenses.

Holding a book close to the eyes will harm vision

Most students with low vision hold materials/books very close. While holding, the book very close to eye, often only one eye is used for reading. This techniques allows the student to read smaller print sizes and is a simple method of magnifying material.

Sight can be conserved

In the past, students with low vision were encouraged to 'save' vision by closing the eyes with cloth/blind folder. It was believed that this would conserve 'the life' of the child's vision. This has been proved untrue. The low vision children should be encouraged to 'use vision' as much as possible. This is in line with the saying: 'if you don't use it, you lose it'.

Sitting close to television will harm the eyes

If a television is working perfectly, vision should not be affected. There is, however, some research being undertaken overseas on the possible effects of VDUs, television etc. on students with low vision. The research relates to length of exposure and proximity of the eyes to the screen.

Dim light will harm the eyes

With some eye conditions, a student may require dim lighting to function more effectively. For example the albino child may need dim or appropriate lighting due to photphobia. Other conditions require additional' lighting.

Loss of vision in one eye severely affects visual functioning

While there is loss of vision on the affected side and a general loss of depth perception, the visual field loss is not reduced by half. Close one eye, look at an object directly in front and see the range of vision which one eye covers.

Chapter II

Assessment of Vision

Low vision assessment aims to document and quantify residual visual function and residual acuity both distance and near, visual field, contrast sensitivity, impact of glare, refraction and colour vision. Educators and rehabilitation professionals may not understand the eye report of a low vision person prescribed by an ophthalmologist. Based on the eye report functional vision assessment must be carried out. Hence it is considered essential to understand the eye report.

What is Low Vision?

Low vision is a term used to describe varying degrees of vision loss, but not total blindness. Low vision is caused by disease, trauma or a congenital disorder. Vision loss may be due to:

- Decreased visual acuities - (can identify only larger sized objects at a specific distance).
- Visual field defects (contraction of the visual area seen, or defects within the normal span of vision).

- Decreased contrast sensitivity (reduced ability to discriminate an object against a similarly - coloured background)
- Loss of colour perception or commonly two or more of the above mentioned causes.

Vision assessment is an important part of the medical care of children. Severe visual abnormalities, for example, cataracts (a clouding that develops in the crystalline lens of the eye obstructing the passage of light) strabismus (squint eyes preventing proper binocular vision) etc. that are not treated in the first few months or years of life can lead to the development of amblyopia or lazy eye.

Visual Development

The visual system which includes retina, optic nerves and visual cortex is immature at birth. It begins to mature during the first weeks of life. Myelination of the optic nerves, development of visual cortex and the lateral geniculate body occur over the first two years. Myelination is a process closely associated with the development of the functional capacity of neurons. One of its chief characteristics is the promotion of impulse conduction, which enhances the functional efficiency of the neurons. Neurons are capable of rapid transmission. Optic nerve fibres begin to show early myelination at birth and will be completed by the end of the third month including optic tracks, lateral geniculate body (it is a sensory relay nucleus in the thalamus of the brain), optic radiations and visual cortex. The visual cortex is the place where objects in and out of their visual cortex is analyzed in detail. The visual cortex is the most massive system in the human brain and is responsible for processing the visual image. It lies at the rear of the brain. For analysis of form, there are cells that respond to wavelengths coming from an object in relation to wavelengths from objects in other parts of the filed of view. The visual cortex is the first location in which signals from two eyes converge into a single cell. Visual cortex is the first location where one finds cells sensitive to disparity, that is, cells responding to objects nearer than the point of fixation and cells responding to objects further than the point of fixation (Poggio, Gonzalex and Krause, 1998).

The fovea, the most visually sensitive part of the retina, reaches maturity at approximately four years of age.

The period of visual maturation is a crucial period during which the visual system is affected by outside influences. Visual stimuli are critical to the development of normal vision.

Development of the visual pathways in the central nervous system requires that the brain receive equally clear, focussed images from both eyes. Any occular process for example refractive error, strabismus or squint eye, cataract, the cloudiness of the lens etc that interferes with or inhibits the development of the visual pathways may result in amblyopia. Amblyopia is a functional reduction in the visual acuity of an eye caused by disuse or misuse during the critical period of visual development. Thus visual behavior and performance evolve with maturation of the visual system.

Vision Assessment

The low vision assessment is usually conducted by an ophthalmologist or optometrist. Ophthalmologists are a doctor's of medicine. They have an in-depth knowledge and understanding of how the whole body works as well as specific knowledge of the function and treatment of the eye. Optometrists have the right training to examine eyes and diagnose vision problems, eye diseases and other conditions. They have in-depth knowledge of disorders of the visual system, the eye and its associated structures. Assessment of vision and prescription of low vision devices are part of a comprehensive low vision service. Assessment might not lead to the provision of low vision devices but will add important information for the person with low vision, their family, eye health workers, educators and rehabilitation workers for planning programmes.

Ophthalmologist's main concern is the health of the eye. A medical assessment looks for signs of disease or trauma. A medical assessment can offer valuable inferences about function, treatment and surgery. Optometrists bridge the gap between the medical and rehabilitative fields. They are trained to diagnose medical problems. Optometrists often work in cooperative practices with medical practitioners. They also work with educators and rehabilitation specialists to address visual disability. They diagnose and treat body systems related to vision system, for example, retraction.

Low vision assessment endeavours to document and quantify residual visual function and residual functional vision. This helps to identify priority tasks for rehabilitation plans tailored for the individual.

A formal low vision assessment is highly specialized and requires specific skills and sophisticated equipment and devices. It involves assessment of residual acuity both distance and near, visual field, contrast sensitivity, impact of glare, refraction, colour vision etc., Let us discuss the areas one by one.

Distance visual acuity

It is measured with traditional Snellen test or LogMar (Logarithm of the minimum angel of resolution). In a LogMar test the 'steps' between each size are the same throughout the test.

Other tests use the logarithmic principle of regular steps in size but have been produced as single letters or group of letters, numbers or symbols on cards. The directional E and LH symbols can also be used when letters or numbers cannot be named.

LH symbol card

Near visual acuity

Near vision should be tested in all persons with low vision. Near and distance visions are not always to the same degree in all eye conditions. In children, near vision is often not as severely affected as distance vision. The purpose in testing near vision is to determine if the person can cope with near tasks; if they need some changes to the task or the environment; or if spectacles or low vision devices would be useful.

Near vision can be tested using passages of print in LogMar format but if this is not available, letters, numbers and symbols can be used. The smallest print read is the near vision of the individual.

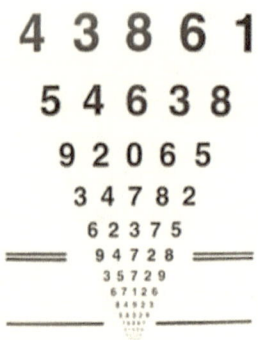

LogMar near vision chart

Contrast sensitivity

It is the ability to detect objects at low contrast. Contrast sensitivity is usually tested with letters, numbers or symbols at standard or intermediate distances.

When there is good contrast with the background, things are easier to see. For example, coffee in a white colour cup. Examples of poor contrast are animals which are the same or similar colour to their environment. For example, view of potato in a white bowl is poor contrast. The following chart diagram shows the high and poor contrast letter.

High contrast			**Poor contrast**		
6	3	2	8	9	7
7	4	1	3	6	4
9	5	8	5	2	1

Similarly, people with eye disease causing low vision are often severely affected by glare. Vision should be tested under various levels of lighting to determine if filters are needed to reduce glare.

Refraction

Refraction is an essential part of low vision assessment to ensure the most appropriate correction of refractive errors. Most low vision devices are used in conjunction with refractive correction. Once clinical assessment made, the low vision child may be referred to functional vision assessment.

The Function of Vision

Vision is functional if a child is able to utilize visual information to plan and carry out a task. For example, if a child sees a red ball lying in the green grass and can locate that ball and successfully pick it up, the child is using vision functionally. Vision is responsible for 80 to 90% of what a child learns during the first six years of life. If visual system (e.g the eye and brain) is not working properly, then the child will need to be instructed how to use vision. The first step in helping a child to learn to use vision is determining how the child now uses the vision he or she has.

What is functional vision assessment?

The functional vision assessment is a method of gathering information about an individual's functional use of vision for the usual tasks of daily life. A functional vision assessment measures how well a child uses vision to perform routine tasks in different places and with different materials throughout the day. The functional vision assessment for example 'paint a picture' activity will provide the information of how a child uses vision and what visual skills the child needs to develop further

The assessment can be conducted in both clinical and non-clinical settings like home, school, community and a rehabilitation centre.

If the individual has prescription eyeglasses, it is important that the eyeglasses be in place during the assessment whenever possible.

The functional vision assessment usually considers the following areas: visual field use, functional acuity, visual pursuit, eye-hand use, colour/pattern/ contrast considerations and lighting needs. As a result of the assessment, the individual's current visual parameters can be better understood and appropriate interventions that reflect strengths and needs can be designed.

Information for the assessment is gathered through a variety of sources and may include input from family members, care providers and educators.

The functional assessment might include a combination of formal and informal screening activities, tools, materials and tasks.

How is a functional vision assessment conducted?

Many items need to be considered in the process of completing a functional vision assessment, but there is a no standard way, since each child and every environment is different. It is crucial to assess the child in everyday settings, doing his or her used activities and tasks.

Assessment of the child's use of visual skills:

- **Visual acuity** at distance with and without correction - with correction means use of eye glasses if prescribed and without correction means visual acuity without using eye glasses
- **Visual acuity** at near distance with and without correction
- **Visual fields** - seeing objects to the sides, above or below the eye level

This test can be done when you think the person may have restricted peripheral visual fields. The person may have difficulty seeing objects to the side, above or below eye level.

In the assessment of visual field, we measure the peripheral visual field by confrontation techniques. Confrontation visual field may be measured by using the tester's finger movement as the stimulus or white or black stripe on a thin stick. The object or fingers are moved towards from behind the person's head and the person tells when he/she sees the object or the finger. An other simple procedure of testing visual field is described below:

According to the height of the person, sit or stand in front of the person being tested, half a metre away and at the same eye level. Ask the person to keep watching your eyes. Hold your arms outstretched at each side and to the front of the person. Ask the person to point to your hand when he sees your fingers moving or keep an object in both hands. In turn move the fingers or object in your hand on your right then left hand. Gradually move both hands inwards towards his face. Stop moving your hands inwards when the person tells that he can see your finger moving. Record the position in the visual fields when he first noticed your fingers moving. Was it at the edges of the peripheral fields or closer to the centre? It is important that he keeps watching your eyes during the test.

Repeat the procedure in the vertical and diagonal directions. All areas of visual field need to be checked. Note if any part of the fields is reduced. Describe the amount of loss as being slight, moderate or significant. Name the part of the fields that is reduced - to the right or left, upper or lower. Depending on the missing part of the visual field the person may have difficulty with objects to the sides, top or low down. Explain to the person how much of the field is missing and show him how he/she can move the head or eyes to look around for objects that could not be seen if he looked straight ahead.

Localizing - spotting or finding the visual stimulus

This can be tested by presenting penlight or coloured plastic strips at about 15 cm in front of child's face. Pupils in the eyes should constrict and the child will pick light on and off to get attention. We can also provide different colored lights.

Fixating - maintaining gaze directly on the object, person or event. Simple activities can be provided to test child's visual fixation. Face the child with group of familiar objects in a tray or in your lap. Pick up one object say a pair of scissors and hold it in different angles. Position it within reach and observe whether the child is fixating. While the child is fixating, pick up another object for example a model car. Hold it in different position. Then present the child with two objects at the same time and ask the child to choose. Children with nystagmus (involuntary movement of the eye) acquire the skill of moving the head rather than eyes through fixation movements when seeing objects or reading.

Scanning - systematically examining an area when completing a task. It helps the ability to search for a particular visual stimulus among other visual stimuli.

Place the objects in front of the child at desk level, and note whether he or she searches in a line from one object to another. Place objects within child's best field of view. Experiment with central and peripheral fields.

An other activity is picking out numbers or letters. Note the following figures. Here figures are superimposed one on the other partially but not completely. Letters or numbers are placed in different parts of the design made by the superimposition. The child is asked to pick out the numbers in one or both of the figures.

e.g

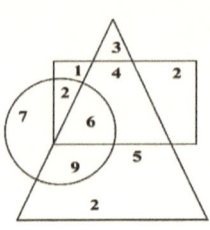

1. Which numbers are in the circle?
2. Which numbers are in the circle but not in the rectangle?
3. Which numbers are in triangle but not in rectangle?
4. Which number is in triangle, rectangle and circle?

Tracking - following the movement of an object, person or event. This is to test how efficiently the child tracks an object visually. Can the person follow the movement of objects without 'losing' where they have gone? In the figure shown, the child is tracking the ball rolled horizontally. Similarly, vertical, diagonal and up and down and circular tracking is also to be tested. Pen torch or a colur stripe tied to a wooden rod cane be used to assess visual tracking at various directions. Note whether the tracking is smooth or jerky and if the child experiences difficulty tracking across his or her midline.

Shifting gaze - looking back and forth from one object or person to another. Give the child a small object for example a model car in one hand held below the eyes and in front of the chest, stand opposite to the person about 2 metres away. Hold up another object say a bright coloured ball in your hand. Tell the child to fixate on the object held in his/her hand and then to change fixation to the ball you are holding and then back to the near object in his hand. Observe if the gaze is shifted accurately from one

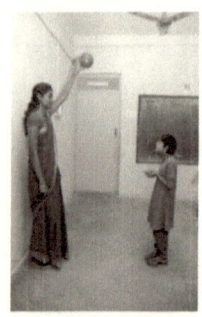

Shifting gaze from near object to distant object

object to another - near, distance, near. Similarly shifting gaze from one object to another can be tested in the following manner. Use two objects (a ball and a model car). Stand 1 metre from the child. Hold the objects in and stretched hands in front of the person at eye level. Tell the person to look at the object in your right hand and then to the object in your out stretching left hand. Show the object and then the other. There should be distinct horizontal eye and or head movement from one object to the other. Repeat the procedure with one object held above your head and other at your waist level. Tell the person to look at the object at the top. Then tell him to look down to see the object at the lower. There should be distinct vertical eye or head movement.

Eye preference - using one eye more frequently than the other. Dominant or leading eye is the eye that we use when we look very carefully at near or at far and can use only one eye. Even when both eyes are used simultaneously one of the eyes is more dominant than the other, as we have hand foot and eye preference. The low vision children due to structure of their impairment have eye preference.

Eye - hand coordination - reaching out to touch something or to pick up an object. It refers to the ability to manipulate objects using hand and eyes in harmony. Activities for testing may include training and copying long and short, straight and curved lines.

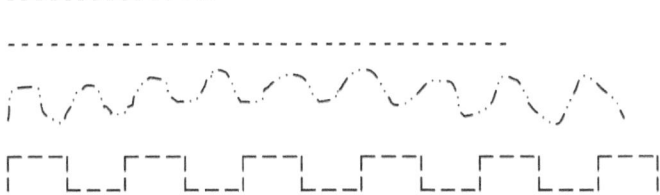

Colour the picture

Fitting geometric shapes in form board, dropping large object in a wide opening and small object in narrow openings, catching ball, colouring the picture, threading beads etc., are some of the activities for eye hand coordination skills.

Colour vision: ability to perceive colour in the context of a functional task. Collect different coloured materials, beads and threads. Include red, green, yellow and blue as they are primary colours. Spread the objects out in front of the person on a table. The table should be plain or with a plain mat. The child can move as close as he wants to see the objects.

Discrimination of colours - Make a group with same colours and same size except one that is different. E.g. Ten blue colour beads and one green colour bead. Ask the child to pick up the different one.

Matching colours - use objects or beads with atleast two of each colours. Pick up one colour bead and in turn ask child to pick the one which is as same as the one held in your hand.

For assessment of functional vision, a variety of items and materials can be used.

Need for Assessment of Functional Vision

This assessment provides information regarding a student's ability to use his vision within the learning environment. It includes acuity, colour, fields, and environmental accommodations. It will include a list of recommendations for modification and adaptations of instructional materials. The clinical evaluation of a student with visual impairment does not always reflect the student's true visual abilities. It is the responsibility of teachers of visually impaired to gather assessment data of a student's use of vision in realistic settings. When assessing a student's functional vision, it is recommended that materials be used with which the student is already familiar and which are at the student's current level of functioning. The activities used for the functional vision assessment should be drawn from a variety of tasks, i.e., academic, non-academic, extracurricular, and social context. In addition to the visual functioning information, information should be gathered from parents and the staff involved with the student. A functional vision assessment tends to be subjective and therefore care must be taken into account.

Children develop visual skills at different rates. The specific nature of visual impairment will influence the rate and level of achievement. In other words, visual functioning is related to the condition of the eye or the structure of impairment. The use of functional vision may be improved with training.

Many children can learn to make better use of their low vision and can function effectively with only small amounts of visual information. Objects and print can be recognized even when they are blurry or even if only parts of them can be seen.

Aim of the Assessment of Visual Functioning

The aim of the assessment of visual functioning is as follows:

- Determine current visual functioning level of the child / adult.

- Determine the visual stimulation and instruction needed to help the person make use of remaining vision.
- Help the child use his limited vision to the highest potential.
- Plan programmes for specific content like orientation and mobility training or adaptive training in use of optical devices like magnifiers, telescopes etc and non-optical devices like reading slit, table lamp etc.
- Use of visual stimulation materials most appropriate to the child.
- Determine nature of the primary reading medium - i.e., whether the child will need to be taught Braille or can he use large print.

Guidelines for selecting objects to use for assessment of visual functioning

The success of an assessment can depend on the objects chosen. So use objects which are familiar and interesting for the child being assessed. Use objects of daily use.-food items, play things which are visually good to use with children. The environmental considerations are very essential which need to be evaluated. They are:

Illumination - Is adequate lighting available? How much lighting does child need given the age condition? What kind of lighting (for example fluorescent or incandescent light) is of great help for the child to utilize his or her vision?

Colour and Contrast - Is there good contrast between the background and the object, person or event the child looks at? e.g Red ball in white background, white rice in a green banana leaf etc,

Size - If a smaller or larger object is used, will the child perform the task easily? Due to limited visual stimuli, it may be difficult to see small object. When the object is bigger, they may not be able to see it at a glance necessiating to see part by part.

Distance - If the visual task is moved closer or further away, will the child see it better?

Time - If the child were given more time, would it be possible for him/her to complete the task better?

Points to remember during the assessment

- Select parts of tests according to what you need to know.
- Allow the person to lean as close as he wishes, or move to look at the material.
- Provide the best lighting conditions that you can arrange.
- Allow plenty of time for each test and encourage without suggesting the answer.
- Use questions like "Where is the basket?"," What is the thing on the table?", "Describe the object near the door", "Do the same as I am doing".
- Ask the child what made things able or not able to be seen. Was it movement, bright clothing, contrast, size, distance or colour?
- Record the actual response.

You can make notes on:

- The objects used for the assessment.

- How easy or difficult - whether the child completes the task
- The child's comments (same, different, cannot see etc)
- Behaviour during the assessment. Whether the child uses one eye or two eyes to see the object whether he sees the object part by part or whole or the child has continuous eye movements/ nystagmus.
- Distance for each item to see.
- The time taken to finish the activity.

Who Conducts A Functional Vision Assessment?

A functional vision assessment is typically conducted by a teacher certified in the area of visual impairment. The specialist is a certified teacher of the visually impaired, trained to evaluate how a child utilizes vision. The vision specialist will measure and observe the visual methods a child uses throughout a routine day and will speak with parents, teachers and other care givers who know the child well. Information about how the child uses vision, the conditions and purpose of use, is essential and will be utilized in the functional vision assessment report. The vision specialist will review records and may talk to the eye doctor to learn more about the child's visual condition.

Interviews

Information from parents, teachers and professionals can be gathered to learn about how the child uses vision during the day. They can describe the way the child grasps utensils, pencils and toys and how he or she moves indoors and outdoors. This information will give the teachers many insights which can be only available from those who are with the child.

Understanding Eye Reports of Children with Low Vision

An eye glass prescription is an order written by an optometrist or ophthalmologist that specifies the value of all parameters appropriate for the low vision child.

The parameters specifies on spectacle prescriptions vary, but typically include the power to which each lens should be made in order to correct blurred vision due to refractive errors including myopia, hyperopia, astigmatism and presbyopia.

Opticians are not eye doctors and therefore, are not licensed to write an eyeglass prescription. A dispensing optician will take a prescription written by an optometrist or ophthalmologist and assemble the frames and lenses to then be dispensed and sold to the concerned individuals.

The prescription typically includes the following:

Spectacle prescription only

For (Name and Address)   Date :

_____   _____

_____

Rx		Sph	Cyl	Axis	Prism	Base
D.V	O.D	-3.75	-0.25	130		
	O.S	+0.50	-1.00	80		
N.V	O.D	+2.00	Add			
	O.S	+2.00				

Remarks   _____
Date of Exam   _____
Dr.   _____ LIC. No   _____

The refractive error or optical prescription is based on two factors:

1. **The spherical (sph)** - This is the strength of the corrective lens required to correct myopia (-) or hypermetropia (+). It is measured in diopters (D). Diopter is the power of lens.
2. **The cylindrical (cyl)** - This is the strength of a lens to correct for astigmatism. It is measured in diopters (D).

Rx means prescription

The eyeglass prescription is written on paper pad that frequently contains a number of different abbreviations and terms:

D.V is an abbreviation of 'distance vision' This specifies the part of the prescription designed primarily to improve far vision.

N.V is an abbreviation for 'near vision' This may represent a single-vision lens prescription to improve near work. Some prescription forms use the '**ADD**' in place of '**N.V**' with a single box to indicate the additional refractive power to be added to the spherical of each eye.

O.D is an abbreviation for oculus dexter. This is a Latin word for 'right eye'. **O.S** is an abbreviation for oculus sinister, a Latin word for 'left eye'. Some eyeglass prescriptions nowadays simply say 'right eye' and 'left eye' instead of O.D. and O.S. Oculus means eye.

Sph: The sphere represents the amount of long/short light that is present. A larger number denotes a strong lens.

A plus sign indicates long sight and minus sign indicates short sight.

Cyl: The cylinder represents the amount of astigmatism that is present that causes vision to be distorted for both distance and near objects. The cylinder may be plus or minus regardless of whether the sphere is positive or negative.

Axis: This represents the orientation of the cylinder (from 0 - 180 degrees) and is the angle at which the lens is set into the frame. The axis is measured an imaginary semi circle with a horizontal baseline that starts with zero degree in the 3 0' clock (or east) direction, and increases to 180 degrees in a counter - clockwise direction.

When cylindrical correction needed, the mathematics used to denote the combination of spherical and cylindrical power in a lens can be noted in two different ways to indicate the same correction. One is called plus - cylinder notation and the other the minus - cylinder notation. These two prescriptions are equivalent.

Spherical	Cylindrical	Axis
+2.00	+1.00	090
+3.00	-1.00	180

Both of them specify a power of +2.00 diopters at the 90th (vertical) meridian and +3.00 diopters at the 180th (horizontal) meridian.

The first one specifies at +2.00 spherical components, which, by itself, would give a power of +2.00 diopters in all meridians, and adds a +1.00 cylindrical component at 180 degrees perpendicular to the axis indicated on the prescription as expanded under axis. The result is +2.00 diopters at the 90th meridian and 2.00 + 1.00 = +3 diopters at the 180th meridian.

The second specifies a +3.00 spherical component, which by itself would give a power of +3.00 diopters in all meridians and adds a -1.00 cylindrical component at 90 degrees. The result is 3.00 - 1.00 = 2.00 diopters at the 90th meridian and +3 diopters at the 180th meridian.

The 'spherical' and 'cylindrical' columns contain lens powers in diopters.

Prism and Base columns are usually left empty, as they are not seen in most prescriptions. Prism refers to a displacement of the image through the lens, and is used to treat eye muscle imbalances or other conditions that cause errors. This is the correction needed to align the eyes, so that they are looking straight and work together. A prism is a lens that bends the path of light without altering its focus. Prism correction is measured in prism diopters. Base refers to the direction of displacement.

In some prescription there is column for **VA** and near **VA**.

VA is visual acuity. Visual acuity indicates the standard of vision when it is corrected. Vision is usually measured using a Snellen chart. You might have seen this chart which is composed of a series of black letters in rows, on a white board as shown in the figure.

Visual acuity is represented as a fraction

Acuities:

- First line   6/60
- Second line   6/36
- Third line   6/24
- Fourth line   6/18
- Fifth line   6/12
- Sixth line   6/9
- Seventh line   6/6

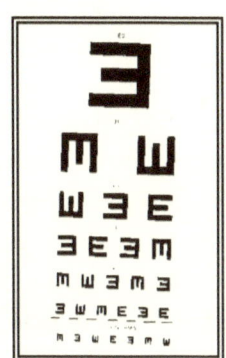

This chart is typically used by optometrists. The chart is viewed at 6 meters. A visual acuity of 6/9 indicates that the chart was viewed at 6 metres and that the lowest line that could be read was labeled 9. Someone with normal vision would be able to read these letters at 9 metres. 6/60 vision indicates that someone could only see the top letter on the chart at 6 metres and that someone with normal vision would be able to read this letter at 60 metres.

Near **VA** - This represents the smallest sized print that can be read with the prescription - N5 is typically the smallest sized type and N8 is approximately the size of news print.

Since vision changes can occur without notice, eye examinations are recommended on regular basis. The minimum recommended frequency of examination for those at low risk for vision as recommended by the Canadian Association of Optometrist (2003) is as follows:

- Infants and toddlers (birth to 24 months) - initial exam at or before six months of age.
- Pre school (2 to 5 years) - at age 3, and prior to entering primary school.

- School age (6 to 19 years) - annually
- Adult (20 to 64 years) - every one to two years.
- Older adult (65 years and older) - annually

A comprehensive eye examination evaluates general eye correction and may result in a correction lens prescription, if appropriate. A number of tests may be conducted to examine the external and internal marks of vision system including eyelashes, eyelids, conjunctiva, iris, lens, cornea, pupils, extraocular muscle, blood vessels, optic nerve and retina.

RECORD FORM
Functional Vision Assessment

Name   :

Age   :

Address / School   :

Vision Assessment   :   Without   With

Distance acuity   correction   correction

Right eye   :

Left eye   :

Both eyes   :

Near acuity   :   Large   Medium   Small
                                N48   N20   N8

Visual field   :

                        Normal / restricted

                        It restricted, describe visual fields.

Contrast   :   ☐ High   ☐ Medium   ☐ Low

Colour discrimination   :

☐ Discriminating colours   ☐ Matching colours

☐ Sorting colours

Additional tests: (give descriptive wherever necessary)

Visual awareness: Ability to spot and find visual stimulus.

Visual fixation:

Is directing the eyes to a particular object or part of it?

Visual scanning:

Is he searching for one or more objects from the background?

Is he accurately moving eyes from one object to another?

Visual tracking:

Can he visually follow the movement of objects without 'losing' where they have gone?

(Different directions of movements should be tested: up and down, side to side, diagonal and forward and back).

Shifting gaze:

- Can he shift gaze from one object to another?
- Is there distinct horizontal eye or head movement?
- Is there distinct vertical eye or head movement?
- Is he changing fixation between near and far object?

Eye hard co ordination:

- Does he manipulate concrete objects using eyes and hands in harmony?
- Is he catching ball?
- Is he hitting ball with hand or bat?

- Is he colouring the picture?
- Is he drawing a crude circle?

Any other remark

Signature of the teachers/Rehabilitation Professional

CHAPTER III

Visual Efficiency

**"Let the child look and look again, and
help him understand what he sees"**

Bill Brohier
Past President International Council for
Education of People with Visual Impairment

The above statement insists that low vision children should be encouraged to use their remaining vision. The use and training of vision is one of the most important aspects of plus curriculum offered by students with low vision. Vision is a learned skill. The development of visual ability is not innate or automatic. Therefore, visual efficiency and coping strategies must be developed from an early age. Functional vision assessments must also be regularly updated since many visual conditions are not static. Visual ability and efficiency can be learned through a sequential programme of visual experiences.

Status of Low Vision Children - A Review

Santhanaraj. V (1999) conducted a study on 650 children labelled as 'blind' studying in residential and integrated schools in South India and Sri Lanka, and found that 40% of them have low vision. While the educational service for blind is more than 100 years old, the education of low vision is of recent origin in developing countries. In the early 1980s, education of low vision was provided with non-visual methods. Teachers of the visually impaired were of the opinion that any child enrolled under the programme for education of the visually impaired should learn special skills like Braille, a tactual medium of learning. When a low-vision child finds it cumbersome to learn through the tactual method, teachers would go to the extent of blindfolding (cover the eyes with a cloth folder) the child and teaching the special skills by touch.

The definition of low vision defined by the World Health Organization and International Council for Education of Children Visually Handicapped conference (WHO-ICEVI) on the 'Management of Low Vision in Children' (1992) is: "A person with low vision is one who has impairment of visual functioning even after treatment and/or standard refractive correction, and has a visual acuity of less than 6/18 to light perception, or a visual field of less than 10^0 from the point of fixation, but who uses, or is potentially able to use vision for planning and/or execution of a task." This is a functional/ working definition of low vision. It recognises that people with limited amounts of vision are low vision. Hence comprehensive services are required to make the child use his vision for day today activities.

Importance of Clinical Evaluation
Unless the impairment is diagnosed very early, the child may miss a great deal of information that contributes to his/

her overall perceptual development. On the other hand, if the impairment is diagnosed, but no effort is made to help the child learn to look in order to see as clearly as possible, perceptual development may again be affected. In developing countries like India, the concept of low vision is not yet fully understood by ophthalmologists/eye care specialists, which prevents them from doing much for functional vision assessment as part of clinical evaluation. The medical report obtained from the eye care centre states only the causes of impairment and acuity readings. This is why the main parts of functional vision assessment will depend on educators/ rehabilitation personnel.

Functional vision is the ability to use vision to perform desired tasks. Because of impairment in the eye and other parts of the system, low vision children will not learn visually without intervention and help. Selection of instructional programmes and techniques requires a thorough assessment and understanding of the child's capabilities. This is mostly done by the educators.

The functional assessment explores how the child uses vision, at what distance he/she sees objects, at what distance certain size symbols can be read, the visual language understood by the child and other educationally and functionally related skills. Observations should be made to determine the technique that the child presently uses in communication, orientation, mobility and daily living skills. After assessment, a training programme should be planned. The training programme includes appropriate sequential visual stimulation activity which would help the child to enhance visual efficiency.

Visual Stimulation

Meaning and Importance

Vision training, also known as vision therapy or consists of a variety of programmes to enhance visual performance. It includes treatments for focusing, binocularity and eye movement problems.

Vision therapy can increase reading efficiency because the goal of vision training is to improve visual efficiency and visual processing. Children rubbing their eyes while reading, avoiding reading, or getting headaches while reading should be evaluated. Problems with focusing (accommodative insufficiency) or problems keeping words single (convergence of divergence problems) may be present. A full eye-health evaluation and vision training workup may reveal problems. Vision training is also appropriate for people learning how to coordinate the eyes after surgery for squint. Vision training can also be used in lazy eye (amblyopia) and includes patching the eye and doing various exercises.

Aims of vision training

The aims of vision training include the following: To encourage and help each child with low vision make best use of vision.

- To provide a variety and a number of opportunities for the child to learn about and understand his environment.

There are three aspects in training for effective use of vision:

1. Stimulation of Vision

Children who have very little vision or have not used vision need to know that they can use their vision. They may also need encouragement do so.

2. Visual Efficiency

How residual vision can be improved through vision training. Measures of vision do not change training-visual acuity, visual fields will not change because of the training.

3. Utilization of Vision

Knowing when and how to use vision leads to knowing how to change the environment/ lighting choosing suitable materials and using low vision devices if needed.

Vision Stimulation: Concept and Procedure

What is Vision Stimulation?

Encouraging the use of vision is vital for children with low vision as it enhances their development, education and experiences. Use of vision in children having minimal amount of vision needs stimulation. Vision stimulation is the use of strong visual stimuli to make an infant or child aware of the vision. These children usually have very limited visual capabilities and no visually guided functions.

Smith and Cote (1982) stated that the area of brain, which is responsible for vision, would remain underdeveloped unless stimulation and visual experiences are provided. How efficiently the child function visually is the direct result of the quality of sequential presentation of visual stimulation experiences. For visually impaired children, the use of vision is not an automatically learned process.

Vision Stimulation Serves Multiple Purposes for Children

- Who have residual vision.
- Who have vision but don't use the vision for visually orientated behaviours or for incidental learning.
- Who have vision but learned to interpret what they see.

The definition of blindness is based on measurements of visual acuity and visual field. These visual functions cannot be measured in young children with the techniques used in the assessment of adult persons. Thousands of young children in our country do not receive early intervention because of the present testing system. Visual impairment affects many areas or development. In infancy vision is very important in interaction-visual communication between the child and the parent, motor development, object communication is the dominant way of communication and visual impairment may affect social contacts, orientation mobility etc. There is a need to stimulate the existing vision to use and to develop assessment of functional vision and define the vision related functions at different age levels.

Activities for Stimulation of Vision

When an infant has severe visual impairment, to help him to learn to see, stimulation must be strong and simple.

Playthings

Toys are more effective for vision stimulation because they are more interesting and easy to use. Many usual playthings are useful. Contrast can be enhanced by adding colours to the surfaces of the play items if the finish is dull.

Bottle with Stripes

Bottles with bright stripes on white background attract the infant to look. Sounds with the water in the bottle may give the child the other source of information-auditory, and may attract the child to look at farther distances. By using different yarns on the surface can give different tactile qualities. Tactile information will be compensatory source of information. The other source of information can be trained together with the use of vision.

Shiny Objects

Shiny surfaces that reflect light are strong stimuli for grasping. Plastic balls covered with shiny papers, shiny papers, shiny rattles etc., which have both visual and auditory stimulation can be used.

String of Beads

The string of beads can be kept in a holder. When the string is brought closer to the child's face the child can grasp it easily. The movement of the beads, its soft sound and the various colours of the beads will be an effective activator in early stimulation.

Illuminated Toys

Illuminated toys and ball or fluorescent ball that glows in a dimly lit room will activate a visually impaired infant.

Flickering Lights

While nothing else seems to work, one may try to use flickering lights at close distance. Because of flicker, the toy can be used by many children with very limited residual vision. The child expresses for the first time the joy of seeing light.

Stimulation during the first month of life and certainly before age six is important for preventing visual deprivation. The presentation of visually interesting stimulus items will motivate a child to become visually attentive. The child might attain visual attention more rapidly provided with an opportunity to experience natural consequences of using vision.

What is Visual Efficiency?

Barraga N.C (1980) explains that "visual efficiency is the most inclusive of all terms... visual acuity at a distance and at near range, control of eye movements, accommodative and adaptive capabilities of the visual mechanism, speed and filtering abilities of the transmitting channels, and speed and quality of the processing ability of the brain are all related to visual efficiency. Visual efficiency is unique to each child and cannot be measured or predicted clinically with any accuracy by medical, psychological or educational personnel."

There are three aspects in training effective use of vision

1. Stimulation of vision - people who have very limited vision or have not used vision need to know that they can use their vision. They may also need encouragement to do so.

2. Visual efficiency - How vision is used can be improved with training. Measures of vision do not change after training.

3. Knowing when and how to use vision leads to knowing how to change the environment - choosing suitable materials using low vision devices if appropriate, adding bright light etc.,

Vision training progarmme

The vision training programme aims to encourage each low vision person making best use of his/her vision. This programme provides opportunities for a low vision person to learn about his environment. Based on the clinical report, vision training programme can be planned for each individual. The functional vision assessment will show which skills need to be trained. For example if a person has some difficulty in tracking an object, training can be given to improve tracking skills.

The following section describes various activities promoting visual efficiency.

Activities to Promote Visual Efficiency

Visual Awareness and Attention

Bright or shiny objects like toys can be used to gain attention. The object is placed in front of the child so that he/she is able to reach and touch it. Start with objects held close to the person. Move the object in your hand and talk about it to get attention. Watch the person's eyes to observe if the object has been noticed. Practise many times until fixation can be maintained. When the person can attend to close objects, increase the distance and hold the objects at different angles in the visual field (front and to sides). Repeat the activity without talking about the object or making any sound with the object.

Activities to develop Eye-Muscle Control

a. Visual Tracking - following a moving object. Hold an object close to the person's face and move it slowly and put it down in front of the person. The movement of the object should be followed with eyes. Hold a light object for example a piece of bright cloth above the person's head as shown in the figure. Allow it to fall slowly to the ground. Ask the person to find it and watch it as it falls. Repeat this activity and watch if he/she sees it and follows the movement. You can ask him to touch it as it falls as an additional activity.

Series of activities such as rolling balls and throwing objects can be provided. A bright ball can be rolled away from the person, then roll it towards the person and then roll it in front from one side to other. The movement of the rolling ball should be followed with eye and or head movement. When the person is able to track the ball, a ball that is smaller in size or less bright can be used as the next activity. When the child's performance is not appropriate, training should be given to achieve the activity. As the child progresses, complex activities can be provided. The person may be trained to track even a rolling mustard seed.

b. Visual Scanning - searching for a particular stimulus among other visual stimuli. Eyes should move smoothly from the first to the second object without going off in other directions. When training in scanning skills start with side to side movement, then up and down and then diagonal movement.

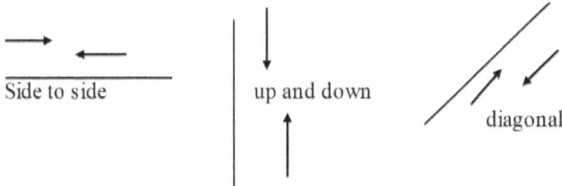

Practise first with the objects close to the person and then increase the distance. Begin with 2 objects and then increase the number. Choose two familiar objects and tell him which is the first object and the second object. Place them in front of the person. Ask the person to see the first object and then go straight to see the second object. The eye movements should go straight to each object in turn and fixate going off in other directions. For example, the first is a model car and the second model basket.

When scanning on sides is accurate, then train scanning up and down and then in diagonal movements.

Ask the person to close his eyes. Place a row of objects on a table or the ground in front of the person as shown in the figure, tell him to open his eyes and ask him to see the object starting at the beginning of the row, and look to the end. Objects can be scattered and the activity can be repeated. Eye movements should be from one object to another without going back to objects.

Give a picture with details about a scene as shown in following two the pictures. Ask the person to describe the scene.

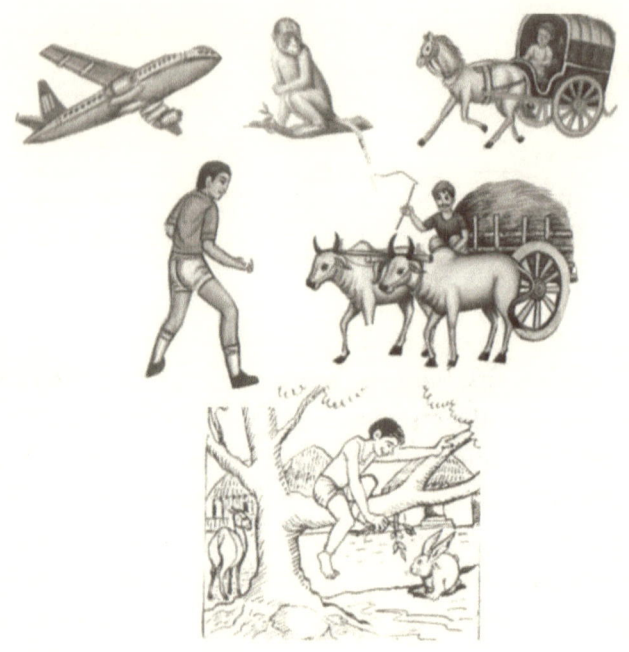

Visual Discrimination

Visual discrimination is the ability to distinguish between variables. Activities for discrimination of colour, size, shape, position and contrast can be given. Colour can be used to discriminate between objects if the person learn the colour of the object such as clothing or food items.

The shape of an object can give clues to identify objects. For example shape of fruits (banana, apple etc) table, chair can give clues and with the outline of the shape, the person may identify the objects.

In the figure shown, the child is given four identical pencils and one pencil without a rubber/eraser at the back of the pencil. The child is given training to identify the one which is different in shape.

Differences in size of objects can help in recognition. E.g an adult is different from a child or a cat is different from a dog.

See the following model cars. Three cars are identical and one is the bigger one. Give such models in 3D or in 2D and ask the child to recognize the differences in size.

Imitation of body movements is another important activity. Start with moving the whole body like bending over or turning around or legs or hand position as shown in the figures.

Large movement of the body

Then large movement of the arms or legs like kicking or throwing and then small parts of the body such as head movement, screwing hand into a fist. Pointing smaller movements with hands and fingers are more difficult to see and copy. Work close to the person then move further away.

Visual Figure-Ground Discrimination

It is the ability to isolate a particular stimulus from the background, i.e. seeing the distinctive features of an object. The teacher can give the child a picture (e.g. the picture of a flower pot). The child can be asked to circle certain item say, leaves in the picture. Models of birds or animals may also be presented. The child can be asked to point out the bird/animal in a group which is similar to the one that is presented separately, as shown in the following picture. Show the picture of an animal as the one in the box.

Visual Memory

It is the ability to store and recall past experiences and integrate these with new ones. Recognizing familiar persons/

cine stars in photographs. The child can be given a picture of familiar environments like the post office, bank, circus, etc. to see for half-a-minute; then the picture is taken away and the child is asked to describe what he/she has seen in the picture. The person has to describe from what stored in the memory.

Visual Closure

It is the ability to perceive a total picture or object when only a part is visible/available. The person has to tell or show the necessary part that is missing in a picture. Examples are people or animals with a leg missing or a bird without a beak or wings. By showing missing parts of shapes, the person has to draw in or point to the missing part such as a square or rectangle with only three sides as shown in the figures.

Identification of whole from partly seen figures

Finding partly hidden objects in picture is an other activity. An example would be an animal partly hidden behind a bush or tree. Identification of familiar person in the picture, assembling known objects from component parts etc. are some of the activities to develop the skill.

Form Constancy

It is the ability to perceive the same object at different angles. Objects like a knife, scissors, comb, spoon etc. can be held at different angles for identification. Pictures of a bucket, chair, etc. can be pasted at different angles and the child should be trained to view different appearances of the same object.

Hard-Eye Coordination

This is the ability to perform a task using hands and eyes in harmony. Activities like colouring of pictures, cutting and pasting, threading beads, fetching a ball, throwing things on the ground, etc. can be provided.

Dot - to dot patterns can be given. Start with 1cm apart from 4cm apart.

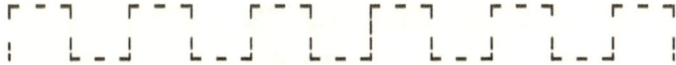

Tips for vision training

- Use familiar objects
- Conduct training as part of everyday activities
- Arrange short training sessions
- Provide a variety of items so that the person does not become bored of the training
- Conduct the activity in a play way method and it can be a fun to the child
- When the child is frustrated of not doing an activity, do not insist the child to do it again and again
- Move to next skill when one skill is achieved. Some visual skills may take weeks or months to achieve
- Not all skills can be achieved by all people. If a skill cannot be achieved, teach in a different way to do the same thing (e.g visual recognition of people by their voices)
- Include training of other senses such as hearing and touch in the programmes
- Work in the best possible lighting conditions

- Ensure that the size of the object and the working distance is right for each person
- Use dark pens to draw shapes and for writing

Principles in training visual skills:

A record of the items/activities achieved should be maintained. While imparting training in visual skills, certain general principles should be adopted.

a. Work from simple to complex
b. Work from real objects and people to pictures
c. Start with actions and sequencing pictures
d. Finally, work with numbers and letters.

Depending on the use of vision by the child, training can be given in stages:

a. By touch only
b. By touch and vision
c. By vision confirming by touch
d. By vision only

Supportive Devices

Enhancing visual efficiency in low vision also involves the use of supportive devices, which include optical devices, non-optical devices and other technology.

The visual efficiency of low-vision persons, irrespective of age or eye conditions, can be increased by a planned programme of visual learning experiences. The most important aspect is that they should be encouraged and

In this Unit we learnt that low vision children should be encouraged to use their remaining vision and the definition of visual efficiency in a comprehensive manner. This Unit described the method of conducting vision training programme to develop visual skills viz visual awareness and attention, visual tracking, scanning, visual discrimination, visual figure-ground discrimination, visual memory, visual closure, from constancy and eye-hand coordination. The points to be borne in mind and the principles in training visual skills incorporated in this Unit are considered important while planning visual efficiency programme.

CHAPTER IV

Learning Media Assessment & Techniques of Teaching Print

Approximately 90% of individuals with visual impairments have functional vision or low vision and just 10% are functionally blind. However, students with low vision are often an overlooked majority in the population of children who are visually impaired. Difficulties of students with low vision are often not as apparent as they are for students who are blind. Students with low vision require direct instruction in literacy. Educational interventions are crucial to help students in any school setting.

Blind and Low Vision Children

In the education of the visually impaired children, there are two main categories -

1. those who use techniques typical to blind persons
2. those who use varying combination of low vision techniques and also blind techniques.

While blind children and their study techniques are rather similar, low-vision children and their techniques are highly individual due to structure of their impairment and the degree of disability. A number of techniques need to be used in all areas of daily functions. Selection of effective study techniques requires a thorough assessment and understanding of the child's visual capabilities.

Screening of Visual Impairment

In screening of visual impairment there are five different groups that are classified for educational purposes:

i.   Person with no light perception
ii. Person with light perception without projection (light can be perceived but not its location)
iii. Person with light perception with projection (location of light can be perceived)
iv. Person having visual acuity of < 3/60
v.   Person with visual acuity from 3/60 to 6/24.

Children in the groups I & II use techniques of blind persons in all these functions but children in group II may use vision in orientation in the known environment. They can discriminate day and night, locating sunlight and they may identify direction. They could identify rooms when the doors are open where light comes out. Children in group III use techniques of blind people in most areas of learning. Although most of them are Braille readers, they may have good use of visual teaching materials if these are relatively simple and drawn at high contrast. Many of them can use colours quite well as a source of additional information. This could be paid more attention since colour coding would be a simple and effective for helping these children to use their vision.

The children in group IV are classified as children with moderate to severe low vision and are functionally very different. Therefore their assessment requires more tests. The children in group V have moderate to significant residual vision. In this group too, each child with learning problems needs thorough assessment.

Low vision is a complex entity. It includes a number of visual problems. Low vision can mean tunnel vision (it is looking through a tube) peripheral vision only (centered vision is lost but only visual intact in the peripheral area), scattered vision (like looking through a broken mirror), depressed vision (things appear blurry) or any number of other visual ailments.

Assessment for Educational Purpose

a.   Distance Visual Acuity

'Distance visual acuity' measurement is the first test performed on the child. If administered correctly, it sets the tone for the rest of the examination. Information on distance visual acuity helps teachers determine how the student can perform activities such as black board, chart and television viewing or physical education. The children can be tested with optotypes including Illiterate E, Landolt C, Snellen chart, or LH symbol set test.

b.   Near Visual Acuity

The major concern of measuring near vision is to involve the children in near tasks especially in reading. There are numerous charts available with single letters, numbers, multiple letters and numbers, words, phrases and sentences with varying levels of difficulty. A suggested starting point is a chart with single words or numbers. If Illiterate E or the Landolt rings are used to distance acuity, they can also be used to test near vision. This type of chart will be easier for the children to see and elicit the most positive response. This test gives a preliminary information on the size of the texts the child might be able to see.

c. Reading Acuity

1. Threshold

This is the measurement of the smallest text size that the child can read at a comfortable distance and what is the smallest size that the child can read at a closer distance.

e.g - The low vision child reads 12 point text at 25cm distance which the child finds comfortable. Then child can read 8 point text at 10cm.

2. Optimal size

Measurement of how much larger the text needs to be to allow fluent reading for a longer period of time (optimal reading) based on the measurement of the optimal size of the texts. The teacher can calculate the size of the texts the child uses in his / her class room. Magnifiers can be provided if the child can be benefitted out of it.

3. Reading Speed

Measurement of how many words per minute the child can read of an age appropriate text and how many reading errors he makes and kind of errors viz, regression, addition, substitution and omission is crucial to develop reading skills.

Reading speed with a minimum of 25 words per minute is needed for comprehension.

4. Reading Comprehension

It is testing the ability of the child's comprehension of the text during the first reading. The teacher needs to prepare a few questions about the content of the passage before hand and the child's answer may be recorded. If the child uses all the energy in reading and does not remember the content, he/she can be allowed for second reading. Finally, the teacher can ask the child about possible distortions of straight lines and about blurred letters or disappearing of some letters to get an idea of the quality of the central field for reading. If there is a loss in the central field of vision, the reading speed may remain low, even after training.

d. Educational Implications of Eye Conditions

The teacher of visually impaired children usually serves children with a variety of eye conditions. A general knowledge of educational implications of eye conditions can be helpful to the teacher of the visually impaired children. So, a teacher needs to look in to the report of the ophthalmologist which may provide information about the causes of impairment, field of vision, prescriptive lenses, prognosis etc. This information will offer the teacher some rough guidelines to the teaching of children with specific kinds of eye problems. The type of eye condition is only one among a number of important factors that should be carefully considered in planning educational programmes for the low vision children.

e. Visual Field Testing

Visual, 'field testing with low vision persons is more of a functional test than disease detection- oriented test. This test will give an understanding of the field of view of the person. The information is used to determine the need to refer to for orientation and mobility services.

f. Contrast Sensitivity

"Contrast sensitivity measurement has been suggested as an important part of the assessment of the patients with low vision, particularly as it may indicate the need for increased illumination and contrast for reading" (Hyvarinen et al.l990, Whittaker & Lovie; Kitchen, 1993).

Proper contrast between the visual task and the background improves visual performance. If the background is too much brighter or darker than the brightness of the visual task, it forces adaptation from one brightness level to the other, with a resulting loss in visual performance.

Visual information at low contrast levels is particularly important in communication and orientation and mobility but also in some near vision tasks like reading and writing.

g. Illumination

Brightness or a sufficient quantity of light is essential to the visual learner to accomplish visual tasks. Most visually impaired children benefit from high levels of illumination. Average to brighter lighting would generally be needed for retinitis pigmentosa, glaucoma, corneal scarring, coloboma iris, diabetic retinopathy, retrolental fibroplasia, retinal detachment, and uveitis. Average to dim lighting is preferred in albinism, aniridia, surgical aphakia, peripheral cataracts, corneal grafts, dislocation of lens etc., Dim lighting is needed with achromatopsia. Glare is any brightness condition that causes discomfort, annoyance, loss of visual performance or eye fatigue. Protection from glare can improve visual functions. Glare in the reading task can be prevented by careful selection of textbooks which use non-glossy inks and paper. Proper seating of the child in the classroom can help reduce glare. The children should sit and stand in positions which direct their vision away from the windows. Pictures, charts, and other visual materials should never be placed between or adjacent to the windows. Natural light coming from top and bottom of the windows is usually better because of less glare.

h.   Colour Vision:

Most individuals with colour vision defects either have less sensitivity in the cones in general or lack pigment in certain cones. The easiest test is to have match colours and sort colours.

Learning Media Assessments

One of the first questions asked about a child's learning is what his/her primary reading medium will be. Teachers and parents may be uncertain as to whether a child should learn braille, rely on large print or use regular print for accessing reading material. The purpose of the learning media assessment is to determine the most effective medium for accessing instruction and teaching methods. The learning media assessment covers both general learning media and literacy media. General learning media are instructional materials and instructional methods. Literacy media refers to reading and writing in print and braille. Let us discuss in detail, the selection of appropriate learning medium for children with low vision.

Selecting the appropriate learning medium for children with low vision

The ability to communicate effectively through speaking, listening, reading and writing to the extent of one's abilities is of fundamental importance in achieving assimilation into society. The most vital component of the total communication process is reading. Reading and writing is of equal importance and value for individuals with visual impairments. An efficient reading medium facilitates literacy and integration into school, learning and work environments.

Choice of Reading Medium

For sighted, print medium is the universal method of expressing language. However for children with low vision the decision regarding the appropriate learning medium is not straight forward or predetermined in any way. Since literacy is measured by the ability to demonstrate effective reading and writing medium, much attention must be devoted to making decisions by which each person with visual impairment will read and write.

Visual Process in Print Reading

Reading is not performed through continuous eye movement but through sudden changes of fixation, fixating a given point in a space, encompassing the surrounding letters. The speed limit of the eye to shift from one fixation to another is determined by the time that brain takes to process the information input. Faster reading is not achieved by quicker eye movement but an expansion of visual field. Visual process plays an important part in print reading. Reading speed is a factor specially affected by visual deficits. The reading speed is influenced by factors like visual functioning, kind of pathology, kind of optical help etc., For many young people with vision impairment the inability to read is the most serious consequence of their eye disease because of the input it may have on learning process. Low vision persons have some differential characters that sometimes teachers do not evaluate. Textual information is processed differently by foveal (central) and peripheral (sides) regions of retina.

Which Medium is Superior- Print or Braille?

There has been ample discussion among the professional in the field as to the superiority of one medium over another medium for students with low vision. However such discussion does not reflect a full appreciation for the complexities and differential characteristics of children with low vision. There can be no predetermined reading medium for all students within an arbitrary category and still uphold the principles of educating each child to his or her individual capabilities and needs.

When children who show a preference for gathering information visually can develop efficient reading skills through the visual channel, the primary consideration should be given to instruction in reading in print.

For students who do not have sufficient visual functioning to develop efficient reading in print, the consideration can be given to instruction in reading Braille.

Some children may need both print and Braille for their education and life situations. The value of one medium over other is not a matter. The important factor is the degree of care that is taken in matching the appropriate reading medium with the child's individual sensory and learning capabilities and needs. The task of the teachers is to provide instruction in learning medium or mediums which will allow the child to became a literate adult, not to restrict opportunities for achieving literacy by failing to match a child's existing abilities with the appropriate learning mediums.

Principles in Determining the Reading Medium

The determination of the appropriate learning medium is but one of critical decisions. The appropriate learning medium is based on a set of fundamental principles that reflect the individuality and learning characteristics of each low vision child.

The following are some of the principles:

- Each low vision child must have a learning medium based on the individual needs and abilities.
- The teachers should be knowledgeable of the child's unique abilities and needs.
- Students with low vision possess a wide range of learning characteristics that are unique in themselves (e.g. reading with central vision, reading with peripheral vision etc.) So no global statement can be established for the total population. It should be based on the individual learning characters.

- The students who show a preference for gathering information visually can develop reading skills in print.
- The students who do not have sufficient visual functioning can be given instruction in reading braille.
- Instruction in both print and braille may be appropriate for some students for he may need very large print for some educational purposes and for a majority of his educational aspects he may be using braille. Some children may use print in day time for short duration and braille for night time.
- Some student may read print but cannot write print. They can be allowed to use both methods
- The determination should be based on the student's unique sensory capabilities, ability to receive information through sensory channels, stability and prognosis of the eye condition. The decision should not be on arbitrary criteria such as visual acuity or legal blindness.
- Each student with low vision should be assured that decisions regarding the learning medium are based on the sensory / overall visual functioning
- The teacher who determines the medium should have professional training and professional judgment
- The professional involved in the education of the children with visual impairment should realize that the children should have communication ability to assure independence, and privacy. The teachers and educational team should have professional judgment in matching the appropriate learning

medium with the child's individual sensory and learning capabilities.

Techniques of Teaching Print to Children with Low Vision

Visual Reading

In low vision services, reading print is the specific goal of the low vision persons. When a low vision person considers reading as a task that may occur even as close as half an inch from the eyes.

The test is to differentiate between:

- those people who can see normal print
- those people who can read large print unaided
- those people who require magnification devices or are able to read very large print
- those unable to read print with magnification devices or need Braille.

Independent Visual Reading:

A child who is ready to begin reading will still need visual training in addition to techniques used in reading. Some of the activities are given here to foster visual reading. Activities to promote association of word symbols with objects and actions pictures.

Activities to promote association of word symbols with objects and actions pictures

Use pictures of previously recognized objects accompanied by appropriate words.

Teach related words to pictures:

Play a variety of games in which children match words to pictures using picture cards and word cards.

a. Affix labels to things in the classroom: The children may be asked to read what is written in the slip and take it TO the place/object and fix it.

Action words can be written on individual cards for the child to choose and act out.

Activities to Promote Discrimination, Recognition and Identification of Individual Letter and Word

Match letters: Present letters in unlike configuration. Unlike configuration is easier to identify. So provide this activity prior to complex activities

p	l	m	p	z

Present Letters in **like** configuration

c	a	d	c	e

Match words

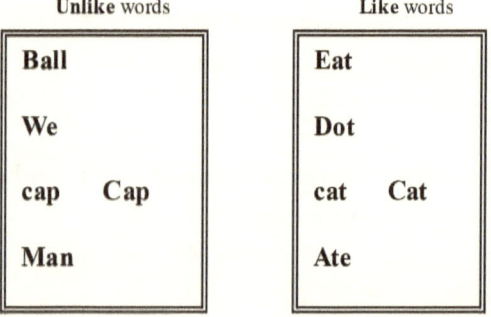

Unlike words	**Like** words
Ball	Eat
We	Dot
cap Cap	cat Cat
Man	Ate

Sort letter cards into proper letter sorting boxes

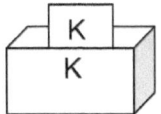 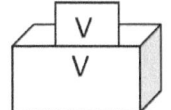 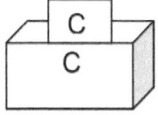

Match letters in work pages:

Identify the letters in the card similar to the one in the circle

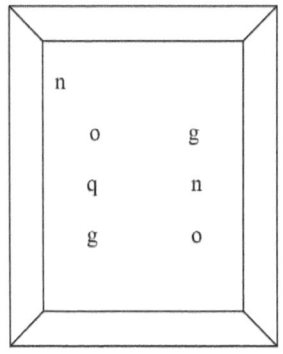 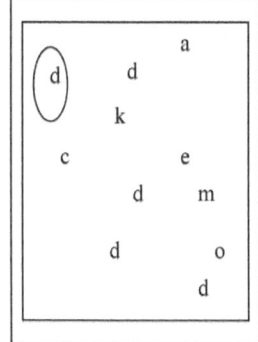

Activities to foster and encourage visual reading of simple materials

a. Use known songs, verses and stories which children can read from memory

b. Make flash cards of words taken from the song/ story (Words from the story) and make the child build sentence.

"Thirsty Crow"

Cow	Thirsty	Forest	Pot	Water

e.g. The Crow was thirsty

d. Begin using text books

e. Provide a story time

Children listen to a short story told by teacher or by an audio cassette. When they have completed listening, the child can follow reading the same story.

Activities to increase reading speed:

The slow reading rate attained by most children with impaired vision is a major frustration. Speed reading techniques must be started early - before bad habits have already been formed. The aim of reading is to absorb the thoughts of the writer, not the single words which combine to express these reading. Reading speed a minimum of 20/25 words per minute is needed for comprehension.

Therefore:

- Systematic scanning technique which develops the ability to spot key words, phrases, sentences, and paragraphs need to be devised.
- Teach children to use principles of continuity and context to make intelligent guesses
- Encourage use of configuration clues.

- Teach children to avoid sub - vocalization which concentrates attention on single words and parts of words rather than ideas expressed.
- The use of line marker / typoscope () offers help to reduce glare and increase contrast and readability.
- Develop good listening skills for more effective use of recorded materials and reader service
- If visual aids are available, develop skill in the use of the devices.

Activities to develop independent writing skills

- Activities for writing can be given simultaneously along with reading activities.
- All hand - eye coordination activities prepare children for writing. These activities should be continued throughout the writing programme.
- Reinforce pre-writing activities before actual writing letters start.

Example:

Some of the writing devices which improve contrast and facilitate writing are:

- Bold-tipped / Fiber -tipped pen

- Black ink
- Line guide
- Bold line paper
- Writing slate used by sighted children and chalk
- Neck-magnifier
- Closed Circuit Television
- Type Writer
- Computer

Teacher Observation Checklist - Signs that may indicate low vision

Teachers in the regular schools may have children with low vision in their classes but do not recognize the signs that indicate that a child has difficulties in seeing. The following list gives some of the most obvious problems these children face.

- Speed of work is very slow
- Working distance is very short
- She or he does not write on the line or between two lines
- Excessively bid or unnaturally small size of written letters
- Partly formed letters or letters drawn in the wrong sequence
- Errors in reading and writing, especially reversals and omissions
- Writing and spacing letters and words in an unusual manner
- Difficulty in copying correctly from the blackboard or even from a textbook or other sources

- Written work does not reflect oral ability
- Confusion in reading certain letters, such as 'cl' for 'd', 'm' for 'n'
- Difficulties in reading long words
- Very slow reading rates, using finger to keep place and guide the eyes
- Consistently losing the place when reading
- Difficulty in searching for information on a page, for instance when using a dictionary or interpreting a graph
- Deterioration in reading after a lengthy period
- An increasing gap between comprehension and reading rate
- Inconsistent quality or variations in the amount of work completed
- Difficulties in reading poor quality worksheets or in processing information which is not presented in a linear manner
- Problems with reading back own handwriting
- Poor attention or concentration span, especially when activities are being demonstrated across the room.
- By fixation the head is kept at a wrong angle
- Seems to look at the side of an object he/she is supposed to look at
- Cannot find the object he/she is looking for
- Fumbles over fine hand-eye coordination activities
- Mixes the names of colours
- Often appearing headaches, easily tired e.g. When looking at pictures etc.
- Wishes for more light

- Is over sensitive to light
- Has difficulties with orientation
- Triples over or bumps into objects, get easily lost, moves carefully and anxiously, has difficulties when walking up/down stairs

Psychosocial Issues

Another issue relating to low vision is the psychosocial impact of a visual impairment. Children growing up with a visual impairment can experience many negative consequences including:

- feeling like they look different, either because they cannot visually verify how others look or because they wear glasses or use optical devices,
- feeling like an outsider because they cannot take part full in activities,
- feeling less than capable because they do not understand visual concepts fully,
- feeling clumsy because they drop things or bump into objects.

All of these consequences can have the effect of lowering self-esteem. It is important that students identify themselves not by their visual impairment but see their visual impairment as one aspect of who they are. Intervention may be necessary so that a student can build successful experiences and find activities in which they excel.

Unique educational interventions are essential for students with low vision in order to ensure successful outcomes in the school setting. The following is a list of resources to help guide the reader to additional information on such interventions.

A comprehensive system of care for persons with low vision has clinical, educational, and social components. It ideally starts by locating persons with visual problems and referring them to eye care or clinical low vision services.

Some children with low vision are taught to read Braille unnecessarily. This child is clearly able to see the Braille dots on the page and, with refraction and/or the provision of low vision devices, should be able to read normal print.

The low vision children should be encouraged to effective use of their best vision. This can involve their learning to write at closer distance, to use magnifying devices, or to use creative strategies to determine what is written on a blackboard such as asking a child seated nearby to read aloud while the teacher writes. This training is important, as it enables children to attend local schools. Inclusive education programmes are one way of achieving many of these social and educational components of care for children with low vision.

A major obstacle to the provision of low vision services is a lack of co-ordination between eye care services and education or rehabilitation services. Each believes that the other will arrange for children to come for an eye examination and/or clinical low vision care or ensure that they obtain the surgery and/or spectacles needed.

It is vital for staff in eye units to ensure that children with low vision are treated and managed appropriately. In situations where the eye care service provider is unable to do this, education programmes must take responsibility.

Caregivers, schools programmes and community-based rehabilitation programmes often give cost as a reason for a child not receiving the clinical components of low vision care. However, transport costs, hospital fees, and the cost of a pair of glasses compare well to the long-term costs of interventions, such as enlarging print using photocopiers, the use of Braille, and education in a special school, for children who may not actually need them.

So it is crucial that eye care providers, community workers, and teachers should firstly direct their efforts towards organising access to eye care, then towards providing surgical and optical interventions, and lastly towards determining what educational support is needed by a child with low vision.

CHAPTER V

Classroom Management

What the Teacher Should Know About Vision

What is it?

Many factors influence how students with vision impairments function in their environment. Some are specifically related to the student while others are external. An awareness of these factors will help the teacher provide opportunities for the student with low vision to perform to maximum potential.

The teacher should liaise with the special teacher who can help by providing more information on the following:

- Eye condition: the degree of damage to the structure of the eyes affects the ability to see objects at distance and near.
- Exposure to visual stimuli provides opportunities to experience and explore with confidence.
- Expectations: parental and teacher expectations plays vital role in developing attitudes toward using vision and low vision aids.

- Encouragement: develops a positive environment which is transferred to the student and the peer group.
- Intrinsic characteristics: each student has individual strengths and difficulties which can affect visual performance.
- Motivation: a motivated student approaches visual tasks with confidence.

Distance vision

Seek advice from parents or special teacher to determine each child's needs.

Visual acuity is a measure used by the medical profession to describe the ability of the eye to perceive the shape of objects in a direct line of Vision.

A student with a visual acuity of 6/60 needs to be at a distance of six metres to identify the standard test type which a person with normal sight can identify at a distance of 60 metres. (Visual acuity of 6/6 is normal vision.)

Distance visual acuity of most students with low vision who receive support from the Department of Education falls within the range of 6/18 to 6/120.

Near vision

Information on distance visual acuity helps classroom teachers determine how the student can perform activities such as blackboard, chart and television viewing or physical education. A measure of near vision is also necessary to establish the size of print suitable for each student with low vision.

Most students with low vision hold material at closer distances than do their peers with normal sight. Some students with conditions which particularly affect their central vision hold material so close that they read with only one eye. Some wear glasses or use other magnifying aids, while aids are of no assistance to others.

A few students require enlargement of some of their reading materials. Teachers trained in vision impairment can help class teachers to interpret data on individual students.

When choosing reading material, it is important to know the near visual acuity measurement of the student with low vision. Almost 90 per cent of students assessed at the Paediatric Low Vision Clinic could see the equivalent of N5-NB print. This near acuity measurement is a guide to visual potential. Most school texts are larger than NB, but for efficient and comfortable reading, it may be necessary to experiment with print size and format for each student.

Some examples of print size are shown below:

SIZE	FOUND IN	EXAMPLE
N40	Sub-headlines	**Most**
N20	Some large-print books	students
N16	Children's books	**with**
N12	Books (texts)	**low**
N10	Magazines, books, texts	vision
N8	Newspapers	can
N6	Telephone books	see
N5	Small ads, bibles	N5 N8 size print

Adapted from Kitchin, J.E. 1985, Management of Low Vision Patients Lecture Manual Department of Optometry, Queensland University of Technology, P.48.

Teacher's Checklist

Teachers are good observers and the signs indicated in the following checklist describe conditions and behaviours which may indicate a visual problem. If observation of clusters of these symptoms demands further action, the school should report any concerns to the parents. Checklist given below is the open source from the Australian Optometrical Association which can be used for identifying signs.

(A) Appearance of eyes

☐   1.   One eye turned in or out

☐   2.   Frequent blinking

☐   3.   Squints or screws up eyes

☐   4.   Red eyes or lids, crusting on lids

☐   5.   Frequent styes or infections

☐   6.   Excessive eye movements

☐   7.   Excessive watering of eyes or light sensitivity

(B) Behaviour

☐   8.   Holds book very close

☐   9.   Avoids close work

☐   10. Loses place when reading, skips lines

☐   11. Omits words or makes errors when reading or copying

☐   12. Closes or covers one eye when reading or doing near work

☐   13. Confuses similar words, fails to recognise same word in different context

☐   14. Has a short attention span when reading or writing

☐   15. Has a poor or unusual sitting posture when reading

☐   16. Tilts head excessively to one side, up or down

☐   17. Makes excessive head movements when reading

☐   18. Squints or frowns to see blackboard clearly

☐   19. Rubs eyes frequently

☐   20. Thrusts head forward to see distant objects

☐   21. Has an obvious tendency to favour one eye

☐   22. Is nervous, irritable, tense or restless after maintaining visual concentration

☐   23. Makes errors in copying at near or from distance to near

(C) Complaints

☐   24. Headaches

☐   25. Difficulty seeing clearly at distance movements

☐   26. Blurring of vision while reading or writing

☐   27. Seeing double

☐   28. Eye burning or itching during or after close work

The Student

Having a student with low vision in the regular classroom requires some modifications to class organisation, teaching styles and techniques. It is important to remember that each student with vision impairment is an individual who will experience the same feelings and fears as other students. The extent of support and encouragement given will enhance the student's ability to meet everyday demands.

For students with low vision, how well they integrate into the class depends largely on their own personality and attitudes; but class teachers can play a major role in promoting positive attitudes within the class.

Some students may be relatively unaffected by their degree of vision loss, but it is difficult for them to remain unaffected by negative attitudes towards them.

Social Development

Because many of the skills used in social interaction are learnt through informal observations, students with low vision are disadvantaged. They cannot watch other people closely and may be unaware that some behaviours are unacceptable to teachers or the peer group.

In particular, they may require help with posture and non-verbal communication skills. It may be necessary to encourage students to make eye contact during conversation and to hold their head up while sitting or standing.

Students could also be encouraged to understand their eye condition so that they can respond confidently to questions and comments they may encounter from their peer group or people in the community.

The family

The birth of a child with a vision impairment puts stress on the family. It is important for teachers to be aware of some of the feelings parents may be experiencing in rearing a child with special needs.

Parents may feel angry, depressed or overwhelmed by the responsibility of teaching their child the skills that sighted children learn spontaneously. They may feel guilty because they have not been able to give the time they would have wished, or they may feel that their other children may have been deprived of their time and attention. Almost all are anxious about their child's future.

The teacher can play an important role in assisting the family by showing an understanding of the parents' feelings and concerns and by helping provide a supportive educational setting.

A teacher who shows empathy and understanding of a child's special needs can help alleviate the parents' anxiety as their child is accepted and participates in a regular school routine.

Parents play an important role in their child's education. Some parents will also be involved in developing individual educational plans (IEPs) for their child.

Ways to Help Low Vision Students

- Find out as much as possible about the child's eye condition. Should any problems arise, that knowledge will give confidence to deal with it.

- Introduce the child with low vision as you would any student. If questions arise, encourage the student to answer.
- Treat the student in exactly the same way as other members of the class.
- Encourage the student with low vision to join in all activities. Advisory visiting teachers can offer suggestions about methods, modifications and aids that may help.
- Encourage the child with low vision to take leadership positions.
- Encourage peer group relationships.
- Use the student's name to attract his or her attention.
- Enhance mobility skills by giving clues and discussing the layout of the environment if required.
- Give verbal clues to make the child aware of events that are out of the field of vision. The child with low vision may not observe a nod, an arm movement or facial expression.
- Encourage the student to use low vision aids when needed and to answer any questions that other members of the class may have about them.

Lighting

The student with low vision will work most comfortably and efficiently where there is good natural light or controlled lighting. Desk lamps may be required in some cases. With some eye conditions, reduced illumination is required and some methods must be used to modify the ambient lighting for one student without detracting from the lighting for the remainder of the class.

In all cases glare is a problem for students with vision impairment, and teachers should avoid standing against a window or in situations where the student is looking towards a source of bright light. Blinds or curtains can be used to reduce glare, and students should be encouraged to wear hats or shades when outdoors.

Eliminate glare as much as possible. This reduces visual fatigue. Shiny desk tops and glossy paper will reflect light and should be avoided. Placing a black or dark matte paper on the desk or tabletop will help to minimize glare and provide contrast. Matte finish paper is recommended for the student's work.

The level of illumination required will depend on the student's visual disability. Some students can be extremely light sensitive. Natural, artificial, day and night lighting present different functional problems and require different solutions for each student. To determine the best lighting, the student and teacher must experiment with lighting conditions.

Aids to control illumination indoors include occluders to improve contrast and block glare, visors to control light intensity and glare, absorptive lens and filters and incandescent lamps. Incandescent lamps emphasize the yellow-red light and have reflector shades and spring arms to help reduce glare and/or increase lighting levels. High-intensity lamps may also be useful. If lamps are used, the light should not shine directly into the student's eyes. Place the lighting to eliminate glare and shadows.

Overhead projectors often have glare. A student with low vision may need a personal print copy of an overhead transparency.

When the student uses the computer, an anti-glare filter screen may be needed.

During outdoors, visors or wide-brimmed hats can control light intensity, and absorptive lenses and filters can minimize glare and reflection.

Contrast

The teacher can increase the amount of information available to a student by maximizing contrast. Sharp contrast between an object and its background makes the object more visible to the student. This is essential in reading, writing, drawing, cutting, pasting and physical education.

- Black and white or black and yellow provide the best contrast. Intense blue, green or purple on a buff or light yellow background may be preferable if glare is a problem. Experiment with the colour of paper the student prefers.
- Keep the chalkboard as clean as possible. The student may have a preference for yellow or white chalk. A white board provides good contrast if glare can be eliminated and a dark marker is used.
- Reduce visual distractions around an object. Avoid using materials with confusing patterns. Keep diagrams sharp, bold and simple. Too many details are confusing.
- Bold, sharp print provides good contrast.
- When enlarging print copies, try to achieve clear, non-blurry copies.
- Bold-lined paper, with varying amounts of space between the lines, may be helpful. The student may

prefer to use pencils and pens with larger points and darker lead and ink.

Desk

Many students with low vision function effectively at short working distances. A raised-top desk or a portable reading and writing stand will help promote good posture and reduce fatigue. If these are not available or the student prefers a regular desk, care should be taken to ensure that the desktop is at the right height for comfortable working.

Blackboard

Placing the student at an appropriate distance from the blackboard can allow for independent viewing.

Generally, the student with low vision is best placed in the middle of the front row in the classroom or seated in the best position for viewing without blocking the view of others. A monocular telescope is often used for reading blackboard work or display materials. When using this aid the student may need to move farther back in the classroom to ensure maximum efficiency for viewing.

The surface of the blackboard should be cleaned regularly and the paint should be in good condition. Writing should be large, clear and uncluttered. Work could be in columns or clearly marked boxes to make copying tasks easier. Yellow or white chalk provides the best contrast.

Whiteboard

Whiteboards is being used increasingly in classrooms. Black or dark blue markers provide the best contrast. Care should be taken when using others, particularly red and green, as some students may be unable to distinguish between these colours.

Similar procedures for setting out should be followed whether using blackboards or whiteboards. Surface glare on whiteboards can cause problems for all students, but particularly for a student with a vision impairment.

To avoid surface glare, it may be necessary to screen off the light source and ensure that students are seated for comfortable viewing.

When extensive copying is required, a worksheet of the work on the board could be supplied to avoid unnecessary fatigue and shorten completion time. Board work and desk work should be alternated to avoid fatigue.

Safety

Students with visual impairments face an extra challenge when travelling around the school building. Most areas of the school present potential problems. Procedures such as drills, changing classes, going to the library and assemblies require that a plan of action be in place. Assess each room that the student will be using for potential hazards. These suggestions will help provide a safe environment.

- Familiarize the student with the school building as soon as possible.
- Limit clutter in the hallways, stairs and classrooms that the student will be using.
- Students with low vision should become familiar with the location of all furniture and fixtures in the room. If furniture must be relocated, be sure to inform the student.

- Highlight the edges of stairs and steps with contrasting coloured tape or paint.
- Keep all cupboard or closet doors closed.
- When going on a field trip or traveling in an unfamiliar environment, arrange for an escort.
- Unless the student is familiar with your voice, identify yourself when conversing with them. Have other students do the same. Always tell the student when you are leaving them.

Seating

The seating in the classroom will depend on the functional vision of the student.

- wwUsually a student with a visual impairment will sit in the front of the classroom to be in closer proximity to the teacher and board.
- If the right eye is stronger, being on the left side of the classroom is best and vice versa.
- Source of lighting needs to be considered. A student with a visual impairment should not face direct light from windows or lighting. The teacher should avoid standing directly in front of a window or light source when teaching to avoid glare.
- If the student uses a reading stand or tilt-topped desk, be sure the desk provides for good posture to decrease fatigue. The student's feet should be flat on the floor and the reading stand tilted so that the student does not have to bend his/her neck uncomfortably.

- For group activities such as story time or videos, the student may require preferential seating.
- A sound field system may be considered for amplification of the teacher's voice and reduction of extraneous noises *as the crowd is more as in the assembly.*

Materials & Equipment

Print materials

Simple typefaces are easier to read.

Density of print, letter spacing, legibility of letters and line spacing are also important considerations.

Use an uncluttered format. Black on white or cream, or strongly contrasting colours are easier to distinguish. A matt finish is recommended.

Colour generates interest, giving dimensional and spatial qualities. Check whether the student has a colour deficiency before using colour combinations as a teaching cue.

Pictures and diagrams should also have a good colour contrast to ensure that the child can recognise and distinguish between details.

Worksheets and notes

When copying work from the board, the student with low vision may not be able to keep up with the class. The teacher can help by verbalising the work as it is written on the board, or by giving the original text or notes to the student. Sometimes other students can provide a copy of their notes.

The best presentation for worksheets is black on white or cream, or clearly photocopied material.

Some worksheets and examination papers may need enlarging. Check with the advisory visiting teacher for the best size print for individual students.

Writing

Writing can be a tiring activity for a student with low vision. As fatigue increases, writing can deteriorate. Although they may try very hard, few students with low vision are neat and speedy writers. Short breaks during writing activities reduce fatigue.

There are many pens, pencils and so on that help the student with low vision. Black felt, nylon or metal-tipped pens or softer lead pencils provide good contrast.

The blue lines in standard exercise books can be very difficult for some students to see. Lines darkened with a black ballpoint pen or specially printed writing books help some students to write more neatly.

Typing

Typing is an important skill for students with low vision as writing can be tiring and difficult to read. Many students begin learning to type from about Year 3 or 4. By learning to touch type through regular instruction and practice, students are equipped with a skill which not only helps them at school with assignments and at home with correspondence, but may help them gain future employment.

With the development of technology many students with low vision are using computers (including laptops).

Some typewriters and computers may have text enlarging and voice output software.

You can get more information about the availability of typing programs, typewriters and computers from the advisory visiting teacher.

Listening

The development of good listening skills is most important for students at all educational levels. As students progress into secondary and tertiary education, greater emphasis is placed on listening.

It is particularly important that students with low vision develop these skills. Commercially-produced kits which are designed to enhance listening skills are available and teacher-made materials will also help.

The class teacher can help the student develop good listening skills by being consistent in giving directions and describing activities the student may not be able to see. These skills are also vital to the development of competence and safety in moving around the environment.

Tape recorders can be useful to supplement some reading and writing activities. Talking calculators are also available. Much of the technology designed for students with vision impairment now has speech output.

Secondary students, in particular, find taped novels a great benefit. Dictaphones are also used for some typing tasks.

An extensive range of taped material is available from Vision Impairment Services at the Low Incidence Support Centre through the advisory visiting teacher service.

Time Modifications

Students with low vision may be able to complete some work as quickly as their classmates, however, they will often experience fatigue...

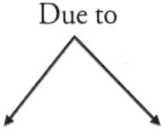

Due to

| shorter working distance and associated postural problems | the need to use a variety of low vision aids |

Some appropriate individualized strategies may have to be introduced.

For example

If the teacher is confident that the student understands the concept or has demonstrated knowledge of content, the quantity of work could be reduced. Five mathematics exercises could be set rather than ten, or three novels read instead of five.

Time allowances for reading tasks should be realistic according to the student's rate of reading.

It may be easier for the student with low vision to answer directly on to the test paper rather than transfer answers to a separate piece of paper.

It has been an established practice to allocate additional time for tests and examinations. For guidelines for a specific student contact the advisory visiting teacher.

Teaching Tips

- Introduce the student with low vision as you would any other student.
- Verbalize praise and disapproval or use gestures such as a hand on the shoulder. Students with low vision may miss the message sent with facial expressions and body language.
- Be specific with descriptive language when explaining the location of a person or object.
- Talk directly to the student, using direct eye contact. Encourage the student to look at you when being addressed or when speaking to you.
- Encourage the student to look directly at people when conversing with them.
- Use a normal tone of voice.
- Feel comfortable using terms such as "look" and "see". They will be part of the student's vocabulary.
- Plan ahead. If a student with low vision requires enlarged texts, audio cassettes or printed materials, they should be ordered or prepared ahead of time.
- Talk while you teach. The student may miss visual cues and written instructions.
- Teach in close proximity to the student when doing demonstrations or using visual aids.
- Verbalize notes as you write on the board. If a student cannot see or keep up with board work, provide him with an enlarged print copy or a scribe to write the notes. Print may be easier to read than cursive writing.

- Allow the student to go up to the board or move the desk closer in order to view or copy the material.
- Check regularly to ensure that the student is making accurate notes.
- Provide extra time to the student. He/she will take longer to complete most tasks. The quantity of work required may be decreased. (e.g instead of 5 math exercises, 3 exercises can be given)
- Consider oral exams or a scribe to write exam answers.
- Use tactile, concrete and real life material as much as possible. This provides opportunities for kinesthetic and tactile learning.
- Sufficient desktop and shelf space is needed to accommodate special materials. The student will need to learn to organize his/her notes, desk, shelves and locker. Colour coding notebooks and files may help. Maintaining organization should become the student's responsibility.
- Alternate visual tasks with non-visual tasks to avoid eye fatigue.
- The student with low vision requires the same discipline and behavior expectations as other students.
- Say, "Tell me what you see" rather than "Can you see this?" when checking if a student can see specific visual material.
- Try to relate new learning to the student's experiences and knowledge. This will help to bridge gaps in learning.

- If a large volume of reading is required, consider having a teacher assistant or another student read the material to the student, or obtain it on audio tape.
- Skip the non-essentials. Older students can highlight important information in print material. Point out parts of the text that can be skipped.
- Provide outlines, point form notes, identify key concepts to help avoid fatigue and frustration when studying.
- The student with low vision may need extra explanation of some materials.
- Hand-over-hand techniques work well to demonstrate certain skills.
- Encourage the student to be assertive. He/she needs to learn when and how to request and refuse help and how to make his/her needs known.
- Encourage independent effort and incorporate proactive measure to reduce the likelihood of the student becoming dependent on others.
- The student's ability to participate in certain activities such as physical education, science labs and visual arts may be affected by his/her functional vision. Modification may be required.

Approximately 90% of individuals with visual impairments have functional or low vision; just 10% are functionally blind. However, students with low vision are often an overlooked majority in the population of children who are visually impaired. Difficulties of students with low vision are often not as apparent as they are for students who are blind. Nonetheless, students with low vision require direct instruction in literacy and functional areas.

CHAPTER VI

Optical And Non-Optical Devices

What is Low Vision Device?

A low vision device is any device that enables a person to improve his or her visual performance. Many people confuse low vision devices with standard eyeglasses. But there is a difference - low vision devices provide some degree of magnification while standard glasses only focus the image for the eye. The use of magnification may lead to some amount of distortion but the image is enlarged, making it easier to see.

Low vision devices are the tools in low vision care. They help low vision persons to acquire functional vision for practical everyday purposes like reading the newspaper, writing a letter, or cutting vegetables and cooking.

Besides using an optical device to magnify or enlarge the retinal image, actually bringing an object closer or enlarging the print can be of great help to the visually impaired persons. These are devices to help to improve visual ability of a person with low vision. Low vision devices may be optical or non-optical.

Optical devices such as a magnifying glass involve the use of lenses to improve vision whereas non-optical devices such as large print help bring images closer to the eyes.

Categories of Low Vision Devices

The two most common low vision devices are magnifiers for seeing objects close at hand known as near viewing and telescopes for seeing objects far away known as distance viewing.

Optical devices or aids use lenses or prisms to magnify, reduce, or otherwise change the shape or location of an image on the eye's retina. Optical devices may be held in the hand, rested on a base or stand, or be placed in a pair of eyeglasses. These devices are called optical devices which involve the use of lenses to improve vision whereas non-optical devices help bring images closer to the eyes. Let us discuss the types of low vision devices in detail.

Optical Devices

Optical aids can greatly benefit some students with low vision. It is important that low vision aids are prescribed by qualified eye care practitioners. One optical aid cannot fulfill all low vision needs and students should be assisted by trained personnel to experiment with the range of prescribed aids to evaluate their suitability for each task.

These aids will not result in normal vision, but will help the student gain maximum visual functioning. Although low vision aids are dispensed after assessment by an ophthalmologist and/or optometrist, teachers can help students use them effectively.

If the teacher has a working knowledge of the aid and its applications and a positive attitude toward its use, the student with low vision may be more comfortable using it. Advisory visiting teachers liaise with the Paediatric Low Vision Clinic and can provide information, training and advice on the use of specific low vision aids.

Optical devices are of two kinds - near and distance. Near devices are designed for magnifying close objects and print. Distance devices are for magnifying things in the distance from about 3 metres to far away.

Optical devices for near Tasks

a. Spectacle Magnifiers

Glasses are the most common low vision aid prescribed. They can be prescribed for distance or general viewing, for near tasks only, or take bifocal form to incorporate distance and near prescriptions. Glasses have the advantage of keeping the hands free. Supplementary lighting and/or a reading stand may also be used to enhance optimum visual functioning.

Low vision spectacles are monocular or binocular convex reading lenses mounted in standard full diameter or half-eye frame. In other words, they are really simple magnifying lenses fitted into a spectacle frame. The convex lens functions to enlarge the images projected on the retina. The lenticular design lenses have less peripheral abrasions. Spectacle magnifiers have stronger and high-powered lenses compared to the usual eye glasses and are designed for close work. The powers range up to + 24.00Ds. Spectacle magnifiers are used for tasks such as long-term reading, writing, needlework, making invoices and receipts etc. They are usually monocular (with the weaker eye blanked out). The person using them needs to hold the reading material very close to their eyes in order to keep the print in focus. One needs some practice to get used to these spectacles.

Uses:

- For reading any material
- Writing
- Looking at objects from close range

Advantages:

- Availability of range of magnification
- Both hands free
- Once used efficiently, can be used for long periods

Disadvantages:

- Exact reading distance important
- Short reading distance with high powered lenses
- More fragile than magnifiers (scratching, breaking)
- Good lighting needed at close distance
- Often a reading stand is beneficial to bring material close

Hand-Held Magnifiers

Hand-held magnifiers are convex lenses mounted with a handle so that they may be held in the hand rather than mounted on glasses. The closer the lens is held to the eye, the larger is the field of view. However, the reading speed and duration are usually slower than with spectacles. The powers are available to 10 - 24 diopters.

Advantages:

- They are generally inexpensive and readily available.
- They are handy for spot reading tasks, in which information is gained from single words or short phrases, like price tags.
- They are portable and provide a variable working distance.
- They can also be used in combination with the person's spectacle correction.

Disadvantages:

- They must be held with one hand or, sometimes, with both hands.
- They are uncomfortable and could cause hand and arm fatigue with extended use. The reduced field of view also slows down reading.
- They must be held at the correct focal distance for maximum power.
- They can be difficult to use for children with limited dexterity or hand tremors.
- They provide a limited field of view in comparison to spectacles.
- They are somewhat less effective than spectacle frames with the same power.

Stand Magnifier

A fixed focus stand is a convex lens in a rigid mount that has been set by the manufacturer to focus closer to the page than its focal distance, to reduce peripheral aberration. Most stand magnifiers are designed for use with a standard bifocal add or reading glasses. Powers are available upto 24 diopters.

Advantages:

- They are handy because the focal distance is stable.
- They are particularly suitable for persons with hand tremors.
- They are especially useful for persons who have difficulty in finding or maintaining the correct distance when using spectacles or hand magnifiers.
- They are useful for persons with a constricted visual field, when held at arm's length.
- They are also available with a built-in light source, which can be highly effective in enhancing contrast.

Disadvantages:

- They have limited mobility, being inconvenient to carry around.
- They are awkward to use on non-flat surfaces; they require the use of a reading stand.
- They have a limited field of view.
- They can cause excess shading and reduce the amount of light on the viewing surface, unless self-illuminated.
- Most available designs make writing difficult, if not impossible.

- Prolonged use of these devices may result in poor posture, unless a reading stand is used.

Optical Devices for Distant Viewing

Telescopes

Monocular telescopes are the most commonly used aid for blackboard viewing and similar classroom tasks, for watching sports, and for excursions. They are particularly useful for mobility. The aid most commonly used is an extra short focus telescope which can be focused from a distance of 30 centimetres. Monoculars can be used with glasses if required.

Optical devices for distance viewing are also known as telescopic devices. They include handheld monoculars, clip-on monoculars, spectacle-mounted telescopes, and contact lens systems. These devices are primarily used for distance tasks beyond arm's reach, such as reading what is on the chalk or white board in a classroom, watching a demonstration in class, spotting street signs, viewing sporting events, or watching television. With training, they can be used to follow moving objects. Some monocular telescopes can be used for both near and distance viewing, such as reading a bus schedule and reading the bus stop sign.

Binoculars

Some binoculars are now available with an extra short focus application. These can also be used for the same tasks as monoculars.

Spectacle Mounted Telescope:

They are mounted on a pair of glasses that incorporate a miniature telescope. This is used for seeing far or near. They can help read matter set at a distance, as when playing music, and are often used for watching television.

Guidelines for Training in the use of Magnifiers:

General Considerations

- Choose a place with appropriate lighting conditions
- Assess if prerequisite skills are mastered, like scanning, techniques for reading across and down a page
- Choose interesting material
- Think of posture and reading distance- a reading stand can be beneficial

Spectacle Magnifiers

- Put them on, while seated at place for reading
- Take book in both hands
- Sit in upright, normal position
- Hold book at arms length
- Move book slowly nearer till letters are clear. The right distance is crucial
- Start reading, by moving the book slowly from left to right in a steady movement, keeping the same reading distance. Rest elbows against sides
- At the end of the line, move the book back to the left

- Move book up slightly, so eyes are on the level of the next line
- Start reading again
- So, instead of moving the eyes, the text is moved. This works for some people but not all. Some prefer to move their head and eyes.

Hand Magnifier

- Place magnifier at the top of the page, at the start of a paragraph
- Ease it slowly towards eyes, till the point is reached where the letters are clearest
- Move head to best position above magnifier; try out a comfortable position
- Move magnifier slowly from right to left, while reading (keeping the same distance between page and magnifier)
- When at the end of the line, move back across the same line to the beginning
- Move down one line and start reading again

Stand Magnifier

- Place stand magnifier (with legs downwards), flat on the page at the beginning of the paragraph
- Move head as close to the lens as needed to get a clear picture and the widest field of view
- Move the magnifier slowly to the right, while reading (keeping it flat on the page)
- At the end of the line, move the magnifier back in a horizontal movement to the beginning of the line

Move down one line, start reading new line. Fingers can be used as a help to locate the next line.

Guidelines for Training in the use of Telescope:

- Find the general direction of the text/tree/etc. you want to look at first, without the telescope
- While looking in the direction of the chosen object raise the telescope to the better or dominant eye.
- Scan slowly to find the beginning of the object (hold telescope steady, keep elbows against the side or on a table)
- If object is text, read from right to left while scanning slowly.

Non - Optical Devices

Non- optical devices include sunglasses, hats or visors with brims, reading stands, dark-lined paper, and black felt-tipped pens. Non optical devices can be grouped according to their function

Devices Reducing Glare:

Glare is distracting scattered light, which is a major problem for persons with low vision. Glare can be controlled with devices such as sun-wear or absorptive lenses, tints and ultraviolet coatings, and anti-reflective coatings.

a. Typoscope

Typoscope or reading slit is made up of a black card board with a slit in it. It is used for blocking out all but the print viewed through the

slit. It should be black so that light from the page will not get reflected. A typoscope assists in finding and keeping the place on a page of print.

b. Felt-tipped or bold tip pens

The larger or bold tip writing pens form larger letters so that low vision person can read letters and words more easily. In order to find the pen that works best for an individual, try experimenting with several different brands and tip thickness until you find one that best meets the writing needs. The writing spaces between lines can range from 1/2 inch to one inch. If you need more space between the lines, try using plain white paper and write as large as you need. If you use plain paper, you can organize and store it in a three-ring binder. You can use a range of three-ring binders to store papers for different purposes.

Filters and shades, hats etc.

With increased awareness of the dangers of exposure to direct sunlight, special care should be taken with students with vision impairment. Sunglasses and hats are recommended when outdoors, and, in some cases, tinted glasses are used indoors to reduce illumination and glare.

Points to remember

- Students need careful instruction in the use of low vision aids.
- Performance should be reviewed regularly to ensure that specific low vision aids are being used appropriately.

- To help students use their distance telescopes effectively, presentation of materials for distance viewing may need to be modified.
- A combination of optical and non-optical aids will be required.
- From the wide range of options available, students should be encouraged to match the aid to the task. (Technology may not always be the appropriate option.)

c. Good lighting on object or print

Lamps and lighting are often the key to improved reading. However, what works is very individual. Some students find reading is easiest with very bright directional light illuminating the page. Other students with an identical eye condition, however, prefer low levels of diffused light. Students often prefer fluorescent lights. Table lamps are helpful for more lighting while reading.

d. Bold lined paper

Bold lined papers with lines that are darker, denser, or wider than regular lined writing paper. Bold line paper can be helpful for low vision persons. Lined paper is easier to write on than blank paper. The lines provide with a reference point for writing letters. We should experiment to find the kind of lined paper that works best for an individual. The students may want to use bold line paper and a marker at first, then move to regular lined paper and a pen as they become more comfortable with writing.

e. Writing guide

Most writing guides use plain paper and a space within the guide frame that provides tactual boundaries for the writing line.

Raised-top desks

Some students prefer a sloping surface for reading and writing. Raised-top desks are available, or portable reading stands can be placed on a flat surface.

Students working on computers or typewriters use a variety of commercially available typing stands which position material within a comfortable working distance.

It is used to avoid back strain or facilitate proper positioning of the reading surface

Large print

You can buy commercially-produced material or enlarge your type on a photocopier.

Writing materials

Use black felt-tipped pens, dark lined books etc.

Electronic Devices:

Electronic devices provide a high level of magnification, excellent contrast and are useful for reading larger amounts of information. There are Closed Circuit Television (CCTV), hand-held cameras, computer programs, and head-mounted systems that allow a variety of educational, recreational and professional activities.

Closed Circuit Television (CCTV):

It has a movable platform for book or paper, a video camera with zoom lens, and a large screen video display. It sets up as a complete system on a desktop. The CCTV reader facilitates comfortable reading and writing at a desk, by people with very poor visual acuity. Some models can be set for any degree of magnification from 2x to 40x or even 60x. Here 'x' means the power of the lens. In other words it is the number of times of magnification. It is also excellent for reading magazines and books.

Portable Electronic Image Magnifiers:

An eyeglass frame is worn that has a miniature video camera attached. It is used for enhanced vision. The camera has a zoom lens which the user can control, and has auto-focus so the images are always sharp. One or both lenses of the eyeglasses serve for both regular direct vision and video enhanced vision.

The higher the magnification, smaller the field of view and shorter the working distance

Computer and Screen Reader

A **Screen Reader** software application reads aloud information displayed on a computer monitor screen. The screen reader reads aloud text within a document, and it also reads aloud information within dialog boxes and error messages. Screen Readers also read aloud and menu selections, graphical icons on the desktop. Recent upgrades are much better reading aloud information on the World Wide Web.

Screen Magnification software enlarges the viewing area of a computer monitor display. Magnification levels are measured in power levels. Such has 2x (2 power), and can go as high a level as 16x magnification. Thus a wide range of software and hardware devices that are available can assist in their education and career avenues.

JAWS (Job Access with Speech) is the most popular screen reader worldwide. JAWS works with the personal computer to provide access to today's software applications and the internet. With its internal software speech synthesizer and the computer sound card, information from the screen is read aloud, providing technology to access a wide variety of information, education and job related applications.

Large print materials

Large print is generally defined as print for text passages that is larger than the print used by that segment of the population with normal vision. The sizes of print most commonly used by the sighted population range from eight to twelve points in size. The American Printing House for the Blind takes the position that large print for use by the low vision population is print that is eighteen points in size or larger.

Larger print is defined as 16 point and over. Evidence shows that many people actually prefer reading a larger print, whether or not they have problems with their sight. Large print is produced around the world for people who have some vision, but are not able or comfortable accessing regular print. Because these population will have a range of eye conditions and as a result a wide variety of requirements, there is no single answer to define large print. As a very rough guide, documents are generally considered to be large print if the font is 16 point or higher. This scale continues up until around 48 point text, at which point individuals may prefer to investigate the use of other accessible format such as Braille or screen reader for their information needs. If you know individuals have specific requirements, the best way to meet those requirements is to ask them. A simple question like "What is your preferred reading format?" can save a large amount of time and money, and is likely to be appreciated by the individual concerned.

What is Clear Print?

Clear print guidelines are '12 or 14 point text in a medium or bold weight, and ensuring a strong contrast between text and its background'. As a very rough guide, documents are generally considered to be large print if the font is 16 point or higher. Because Clear Print is designed to be used for all documents, it has far reaching benefits. A clearly designed and easy to read document will convey the essential information to everyone who reads it.

Tips for achieving clear print

- Document text size should be 12-14 pt, preferably 14 pt.
- The font you choose should be clear, avoiding anything stylised
- All body text should be left aligned
- Use bold sparingly, only highlight a few words rather than a paragraph
- Keep the text layout clear, simple and consistent

- Do not use blocks of capitalised letters, and try not to use any italics or underlining
- Text shouldn't be overlaid on images
- The substrate or coatings should not be glossy or reflective
- Ensure the paper is thick enough to prevent show through
- The contrast between the text and background is as high as possible
- All text should be the same orientation on the page
- Space between columns of text is large enough to be distinct
- Any information conveyed in colour or through images is also described

Guidelines for Preparing Large Print:

American Printing House (APH) has given recommendations based on the researches on the impact of various large print characteristics on reading speed, comprehension, literacy and usability by large print users. The following is the guideline:

Each large print user should have access to:

- A font that is at least 18 points in size.
- X-height and t-heights of at least 1/8 inch.
- A typeface without serifs.
- Spacing between lines of print of at least 1.25 spaces.
- Headings and subheadings that are larger and bolder than regular large print text.
- Paragraphs that are block style and use 1 inch margins. The left margin should be justified and

the right hand margin should not be justified. There should be no first-line indentations to delineate paragraphs.

- Printed materials with no columns or divided words.
- Black print on white, ivory, cream, or yellow paper with a dull finish so as not to promote glare.
- Print that is not used over a background design or other graphical material.
- Graphics that are not only enlarged, but maintain the same contrast, clarity, and appropriate coloration as those prepared for their sighted peers.
- Graphic materials, such as maps, graphs, and charts, which also adhere to type size, font, and other large print guidelines
  1. Full-color or high-quality black line art rather than gray-scale or shaded drawings.
  2. Books that weigh approximately 250 grams and are no larger in dimension than 9 inches by 12 inches by 2.5 inches.

Access to Normal Sized Print - Modern technology has made it possible to access normal pint. People with some remaining vision can use: closed circuit televisions, and large print computer software. People with very little to no remaining vision can use: scanners with optical character recognition software, and text to speech software. For people that read Braille there is software to convert text to Braille, which can be read on a refreshable Braille display, or printed out using a Braille embosser.

CHAPTER VII

Environmental Modification And Orientation Mobility

Environmental modifications are used to improve the independent functioning of children with low vision. The environmental modifications should be provided within the environment where they will be, including home, community, and workplace the low vision devices help the low vision children to use their vision more effectively. While considering environmental modifications, three important features should be remembered.

1. Making things **bigger** and **bolder**

Using a felt pen to write **bolder** print than usual letters may help many low vision persons. Short and simple writing will be helpful due to limited field of vision. Enlarged print making with the help of photocopiers may be easier for the low vision persons to see.

2. Improving **lighting**

Lighting is the best way to improve contrast. If someone wants to read, ensure the page is well lit. It should not shine in their eyes. The light should shine directly onto the page, but without producing glare. Good lighting in darker areas of the home is important, particularly when the person may have fear of going up and down stairs or using outside.

3. Using **contrast** and **colour**

Bringing things closer to the eyes makes them appear bigger. The low vision person who has good accommodation ability may benefit using this technique. Contrast colour may improve visibility. For example, rice is much easier to see in red plate than in the white plate. Colour can be useful in many ways, for example using red tapes around white coloured light switches. To mark stairs, use colored masking tape on the edge of the steps to indicate where the drop-off or step-up will be.

A doorframe fixed on white wall should not be light grey in color because both colours are looking similar. Instead of grey coloured door frame, navy blue doorframe may of greater assistance.

Orientation and Mobility for Low Vision Children

Orientation means as awareness of position in space. Mobility means the capacity of moving around through the environment safely, efficiently, and independently. Not all persons with low vision need orientation and mobility training but those who are unable to move with ease, independent mobility is achieved by gradually exposing them to increasingly complex situations.

Successful mobility depends on effective use of visual information rather than visual acuity. Even minimal visual function such as light perception can be useful. The important aspects in visual functions are influence of visual field, visual acuity, lighting and contrast sensitivity. Of these four variables, peripheral field defect, light levels and contrast sensitivity are more closely related to mobility than is acuity.

Assessment Strategies

The mobility assessment is the first step designing a mobility programme. Instruction may be brief or extended over a period of months depending on the age, goals and abilities. First the mobility instructor/special educator can conduct an interview to uncover problem in mobility related to eye condition and psychological difficulties.

Functional Assessment in Mobility

A functional assessment is very important which is to be conducted indoors and outdoors under actual travel conditions. The functional assessment is to evaluate the child's use of visual information and ability to draw on previous experiences.

The functional assessment includes the following areas:

- Identification and avoidance of obstacles
- Estimation of distances
- Negotiation of steps, curbs and uneven surfaces
- Ability to explore from one point to another
- Lighting needs, and adjustment to variable light condition
- Discrimination of contrast
- Scanning skills
- Use of aids

- Use of inputs in other senses
- Ease and speed of travel

The best assessment is to hear what the low vision person is telling about their needs, desires, problems etc. the instructor should also observe the person in the environment. But keeping those in mind and record, it is more important to analyze actual performance.

Discrepancies may exist between the answers to interview questions and actual performance that could give the evaluator a basis for discussing realistic limitations with the low vision person and designing a practical programme around those limitations.

Training for Adult and Children

The adult does not have to be "taught" to see because spatial concept is usually intact, visual memory and previous experiences are stored. A typical programme for an adult includes training in efficient use of vision and hearing, travel skills in the neighborhood and using public transportation, sighted guide techniques, the use of long cane and use of visual aids.

Children, particularly those whose low vision is congenital or of early onset, need intensive training. A typical programme for a child or young person includes visual simulation, body image, concept development, body movement, sensory training of non-visual senses, independent travel in the known environment, use of visual aids for example use of hand magnifiers to read maps, addresses, telephone numbers etc., and use of mobility techniques such as cane travel and sighted guide.

Mobility Aids and Techniques

1. Conventional Glasses

Conventional spectacle is first prescribed by the eye care specialist to provide the best possible base line visually acuity.

2. Aids that Control Light

The visual aids that modify light, increase contrast or reduce glare includes visors, wide brimmed hats, sunglasses, frames with side shields and telescopes. For persons who are night blind, a bright light source from flash/torch light may be enable the person to travel without cane.

3. Magnification Aids

Monocular telescopes or head-borne bioptic telescopes may enable the low vision persons to localize, focus and track.

4. Minifiers

A person with peripheral field loss can see the effect of minification by reversing a low-power monocular telescope. Minifiers are specially designed to reduce the image size horizontally, which expands only the lateral periphery of the field of vision.

5. Fresnel Prism

A Fresnel prism is a series of prisms compressed into a flat plastic membrane. These are accurately placed on a pair of glasses in the area of a non-functional field of view. Do not interfere with the person's regular vision. The person who is using this, however, with a quick movement into the prism can see objects at the side without any head movement. The prism in effect, defect light rays and cause those objects at one's side to appear in front of the person for easy viewing.

This visual mobility aid is useful for those which severe constricted visual field caused by Retinitis Pigmentosa, Advanced Glaucoma, and less severe case like hemianoptic (half vision) field defects.

Non-visual Aids and Techniques

Some low vision persons may have to use non-visual technique to supplement vision under some conditions such as absence of light, unfamiliar place or uneven terrain etc. Some of the non-visual aids and techniques are:

1. Sighted Guide

A sighted guide technique allows the low vision person to travel comfortably with a companion. Person with peripheral field loss appreciate a sighted guide in poor lighting and a new situation. Older people are often more comfortable with sighted guide.

2. Long Cane

The Long cane, traditionally associated with blindness, can be used by persons with low vision. A person with night blindness who is able to get about easily during the day needs a cane in dim light or at night. A person with a limited visual filed may more freely using residual vision for general orientation and a cane for obstacle and curbs detection.

Protective Arm Technique

The protective arm technique is used to avoid injury to the upper and lower body. This technique is to be used if the person's acuity is insufficient for the occasional situation when no sighted guide or cane is available.

Trailing

Trailing is following a wall or other surface with the back of the hand. Trailing allows a person t o remain in contact with physical guidelines to avoid becoming disoriented.

Adaptations for Optical Visual Functioning

1. Illumination - the amount, direction and changes in lighting conditions are crucial for optimal visual functioning.

2. Wearing absorptive sun lenses which block ultra-violet and infra - red light rays significantly increase functional acuity. In addition it reduces the amount of time it takes to adjust from indoor to outdoor lighting and vice versa.

3. Wearing wide-brim hats or visors, or even using umbrella in the sun help to increase functional acuity and protect one's eye from glare.

4. When trying to discern an object, person or sign, position oneself in such a way that the sun comes from behind the person. Change angle of viewing to facilitate best position.

5. In dim light situations such as some rooms, restaurants and cinemas, use a portable light source such as a penlight or flashlight for spot checking. Appropriate sighted guide or cane techniques are

also recommended in these situations where a person is rendered functionally blind.

6. Depth perception-judgment of presence of drop -offs such as curbs, steps and uneven terrain - is affected not only by the person's reduced visual acuity or fields, but by changes in lighting and contrast.

7. A cane is particularly helpful in these situations as it frees the persons in front of you is helpful especially if that person suddenly appears higher or lower in one's visual field or moves sharply to the right or left, indicating the presence of up and down steps, curbs or uneven terrain.

8. A broken shadow in one's line of path may be indicative of stairs. (E.g., the shadow of pole on a flight of stairs will appear as uneven and broken, not as a straight line.)

Bumping into Obstacles

If vision is always directed downward for safety purposes, using a cane allows freedom to can more effectively and cover a wider path. Following the shoulder line of a person with distinctly contrasting or vivid colour clothing provides movement clues to avoid possible objects.

Learning to visually scan is a systematic search patter as opposed to random, inefficient use of visual skills for visual cues in the environment.

Glossary

A

Absorptive lenses

Eyeglasses with lenses tinted to absorb much of the sun's light and prevent it from entering the eye; sunglasses.

Accommodation

The adjustment of the eye for seeing at different distances, accomplished by changing the shape of the crystalline lens through action of the ciliary muscle, thus focusing a clear image on the retina.

Achromatopsia

A congenital defect in or absence of cones, resulting in the inability to see color and reduced clear central vision.

Age-related macular degeneration

A condition associated with vascular diseases such as arteriosclerosis and stroke, in which the central vision is gradually lost, decreasing in some people to 20/200 or less, but peripheral vision is usually retained. Also called age-related maculopathy.

Albinism

Congenital absence of pigment in skin, hair, iris, choroid and retina, often resulting in defective vision (usually associated with lowered visual acuity, nystagmus and photophobia, and often accompanied by refractive errors).

Amblyopia
Partial blindness, often used to describe the poor vision in a squinting eye (dimness of vision without any apparent disease of the eye).

Amsler grid
A graphlike card used to determine central visual field losses.

Angular magnification
In creasing the apparent size of an object through the use of various lens systems, such as binoculars.

Aniridia
Congenital absence of the iris.

Anterior Chamber
Interior part of the eye, bounded in front by the cornea and behind by the iris, containing the aqueous humour.

Aphakia
Absence of the lens. It is used to describe an eye after a cataract extraction, when the intraocular lens has been removed.

Aqueous Humour
The clear watery fluid which fills the anterior and posterior chambers within the front part of the eye; it is produced by the Ciliary body and drains into the veins of the sclera.

Arrangement test
A type of color vision test that uses color caps to be arranged in a particular order by the individual being tested.

Astigmatism
Refractive error which prevents the light rays from coming to a single focus on the retina because of different degrees of refraction in various meridians of the eye.

Assistive technology
Computer hardware and software used to make the environment and printed information accessible.

Astigmatism
A refractive error caused by a spherocylindrical curvature of the cornea; correctable with a cylindrical lens.

B

Binocular Vision
The ability to use the two eyes simultaneously to focus on the. same object and to fuse the two images into a single image which gives a correct interpretation of its solidity and its position in space.

Bio behavioral states
A range of activity levels from sleep to alert or agitated. The ability to learn requires the maintenance of alert biobehavioral states.

Bioptic telescope
A miniature telescope mounted on an eyeglass lens (called the carrier lens) and positioned above or below the direct line of sight when facing forward. It is used for momentary spotting of objects at a distance.

Blind Spot
A "blank" area in the visual field where there is no vision. It corresponds to the position of the optic nerve.

Blink reflex
A contraction of the eyelid muscles to close the lids that occur spontaneously in response to sudden loud noises, bright lights, sneezing, or a perceived visual threat.

C

Cataract

A condition in which the crystalline lens of the eye, or its capsule, or both, become opaque, with consequent loss of visual acuity; may originate before birth (congenital) or develop progressively in the elderly (senile) or from injury (traumatic).

Central scotoma

Area of diminished or absent vision that result in a blind spot in the center of the visual field.

Cerebral visual impairment

See cortical visual impairment.

Closed-circuit television system (CCTV)

A device that provides electronic magnification by means of a video camera that projects the image onto a television monitor; also known as video magnifier.

Central Visual Acuity

Ability of the eye to perceive the shape of objects in the direct line of vision.

Choroid

The vascular, intermediate coat which furnishes nourishment to the other parts of the eyeball - the membrane lying between the retina and the sclera.

Ciliary Body

The muscles inside the eye that control the shape of the lens and also secrete the aqueous humour.

Portion of the vascular coat between the iris and the choroid. It consists of ciliary processes and the ciliary muscle.

Coloboma

Congenital cleft due to the failure of the eye to complete growth in the part affected.

Colour Deficiency
Diminished ability to perceive differences in colour, usually for red or green,' rarely for blue and yellow.

Color vision
The perception of color as a result of the stimulation of specialized cone receptors in the retina.

Cones and Rods
Two kinds of cells which form a layer of retina and act as light-receiving media. Cones are concerned with visual acuity and colour discrimination. They are responsible for receiving images that are formed on the retina and act in the daylight. Rods are concerned with motion and vision at low degrees of illumination (night vision).

Cone dystrophy
Hereditary degeneration of cones, resulting in decreased vision and a lack of color perception.

Cones
Specialized photoreceptor cells in the retina, primarily concentrated in the macular area, that are responsible for sharp vision and color perception.

Confrontation visual field testing
A method for making an approximate assessment of peripheral vision.

Contact lens
A small plastic disc containing an optical correction that is worn directly on the cornea as a substitute for eyeglasses.

Congenital
Present at birth.

Contrast sensitivity
The ability to detect small changes in brightness

Convex lens

A lens that bends light rays inward and is used to correct for hyperopia. Also called plus lens. See alos spherical lens.

Concave lens

A lens that spreads out light rays and is used to correct for myopia. Also called minus lens. See also spherical lens.

Conjunctiva

Mucous membrane which lines the eyelids and covers the front part of the eyeball (white part). It does not cover the cornea.

Convergence

Coordinated movement of the two eyes to allow fixation on the same point of vision, with the result that the pupils of the eyes are closer together. The eyes are turned inward. Convergence deficiency is the inability to converge the eyes.

Convergent Squint

A deviation of one eye towards the nose, as distinct from divergent.

Cornea

Clear, transparent portion of the outer coat of the eyeball, forming front of aqueous chamber. The front surface of the eye, highly specialised clear tissue which lies in front of the iris.

Corneal Graft

Operation to restore vision by replacing a section of opaque cornea with transparent cornea.

Cortical visual impairment

Visually impairment caused by change to the posterior visual pathways and /or the occipital lobe of the brain.

Corneal Scarring

Caused by inflammatory conditions such as, keratitis, and resulting in loss of transparency of cornea, and hence loss of visual acuity.

Correction

Returning to normal; when referring to glasses, correction of refraction means prescription of suitable lenses to bring the vision back to normal; e.g. refractive errors caused when eyeball is too short (long-sighted or hypermetropic) or too long (short-sighted or myopic) or astigmatism (distortion due to unequal curvature of lens or cornea). Correction of a squint refers to normalisin the angle of deviation between the two eyes.

D

Depth Perception

The ability to perceive the solidity of' objects and their relative position in space.

Depth of field

The range of distances that an object can be from a lens and still appear to be in focus to the observer.

Dioptre

Unit of measurement of strength or refractive power of a lens.

Diplopia

Double vision

Diabetic retinopathy

Range of retinal changes associated with long-standing diabetes. Stages include nonproliferative (early) and proliferative (when blood vessels grow abnormally and fibrous tissues form).

Dislocation of the Lens

A condition resulting from some defect in the suspensory ligaments, resulting in the lens being misplaced or not in its correct position; focus and accommodations are affected.

Distance Vision

Ability of the eye to see when looking at an object in the distance: 6 metres is accepted as standard for clinical measurement of distance vision.

E

Eccentric viewing

Looking to the side, above, below, or above an object of regard in order to place it in best focus. This often is necessary when there has been damage to the fovea.

Electronic magnification systems

Machines that produce enlarged images, including closed circuit televisions, computer systems, and low vision enhancement devices.

Emmetropia

The refractive condition of the normal eye. When the eye is at rest, the image of distant objects is brought to a focus on the retina.

Environmental adaptation or modification

Change in the environment to maximize a person's ability to function.

Esophoria

A tendency of the eye' to turn inward (converge).

Esotropia

A manifest turning inward of the eye (convergent strabismus or crossed eye).

Exophoria
A tendency for the eye to turn outwards (diverge).

Exotropia
a form of strabismus in which one or both eyes deviate outward.

Eye Dominance
Tendency of one eye to assume the major function of seeing, being assisted by the less dominant eye.

F

Field Of Vision
The entire area which can be seen without shifting the gaze.

Figure-ground perception
Ability to discriminate an object visually against its background.

Fixating
Directing the eye so that the object of interest is imaged on the fovea or the preferred retinal locus.

Focal point
The point at which parallel light rays are brought to a focus by a lens.

Form constancy
Ability to identify form regardless of size, orientation, or if embedded in other forms.

Focus
Point to which rays are converged after passing through a lens; focal distance is the distance rays travel after refraction before focus is reached.

Fovea
Small depression in the retina at the back of the eye; the part of the macula adapted for most acute vision.
Functional vision
The ability to use vision in planning and performing a task.
Functional vision evaluation
An evaluation of visual abilities as used in functional tasks, such as reading, tasks of daily living, vocational pursuits for older children and adults, and educational programming for students and most often conducted in the person's usual home, school, or work environment. Also known as functional vision assessment.
Fusion
The power of coordinating the images received by the two eyes into a single mental image.

G
Glare
Discomfort produced by too much light in the visual field.
Glaucoma
Increased pressure inside the eye; "hardening of the eyeball" caused by accumulation of aqueous fluid in the front portion. Progressive damage to the optic nerve results in loss of visual acuity.

H
Hemianopsia
A defect in either half of the visual field. Also called hemianopia.
Henlanopialhemianopia
Blindness of one-half of the field of vision of one or both eyes.

Hyperopia (farsightedness)
A refractive error caused by an eyeball that is too short; corrected with a plus (convex) lens.

I
Individualized education program (IEP)
A written plan of instruction for a student who receives special education services, developed by an educational team that includes the student and family.

Individualized written rehabilitation program (IWRP)
A contract between a person and a rehabilitation agency that describes the services needed to achieve that person's employment objective.

Interdisciplinary team
Specialists who work individually with clients or students, but among whom there is communication.

Iris
Coloured, circular mem brane suspended behind the cornea and immediately in front of the lens. The iris regulates the amount of light entering the eye by changing the size of the pupil.

K
Keratoconus
Cone-shaped deformity of the cornea.

L
Lens
A transparent structure with nonparallel sides that alters (converges or diverges) rays of light.

Light projection
The ability to discern the source or direction of light, but not enough vision to identify objects, people, shapes, or movements.

Literacy medium
The method used by an individual to read and write.

Light Adaptation
The power of the eye to adjust itself to variations in the amount of light.

Localizing
Having an awareness of the location of an objet of interest in the environment from visual, auditory, or kinesthetic cues so that a fixation can be directed toward it.

Low vision
A vision loss severe enough to impede an individual's ability to learn or perform usual tasks of daily life, given that individual's level of maturity and cultural useful visual discrimination. Low vision cannot be corrected to normal by regular eyeglasses or contact lenses and covers a range from mild to severe vision loss but excludes complete loss of functional vision.

Lower Vision Aids
Optical devices of various types useful to persons with vision impairment.

Low vision evaluation
A comprehensive examination, performed by an optometrist or ophthalmologist, that investigates many of the same factors as in a basic eye examination, but also may involve the use of different techniques leading to more precise results for individuals with low vision.

M

Macula (Macular Region)

The small central area of the retina that contains the fovea; with the fovea comprises the area of distinct vision. Synonym: yellow spot.

Magnifier

A device to increase the size of an image through the use of lenses or lens systems.

Macular Degeneration

Disease most common in the elderly, resulting in deterioration of the central vision, i.e. the area of vision used for fine detail: peripheral vision is unaffected.

Minus lens

See Concave lens.

Monocular telescope

A telescope that can be used in the preferred eye.

Myopia

A refractive error in which, because the (short sight) eyeball is too long in relation to its focusing power, the point of focus for rays of light from distant objects (parallel light rays) is in front of the retina. Thus, to obtain distinct vision, the object must be brought nearer to take advantage of divergent light rays (those from objects less than 20 feet away). It is generally corrected by spectacles but extreme myopia can be pathological, causing gradual loss of acuity, resulting in blindness.

N

Near Point Of Accommodation

The nearest point at which the eye can perceive an object distinctly. It varies according to the power of accommodation.

Near Vision

Ability of the eye to perceive distinctly objects at normal distance: 35 cm. is accepted as standard for clinical measurement of near vision.

Night Blindness

A condition in which the sight is good by day but deficient at night and in faint light.

Non-optical devices

Devices or modifications that do not involve lenses, used to individuals with low vision, such as reading stands, trays, positioning and seating, modifications of illumination, and large print.

Nystagmus

An involuntary rapid oscillatory movement of the eyeball, often congenital. It may be vertical, lateral, rotary or mixed. It may be present in eyes which otherwise appear to be normal, but also occurs in cases of albinism, congenital cataract and retinal disorders.

O

Occlusion

The blocking of the vision in one eye, usually in the treatment of squints.

Opacity

Cloudiness. Most opacities in the eye are caused by small cloudy areas in the lens or cornea which do not allow the transmission of light.

Optic Atrophy

Degeneration of the optic nerve tissue which carries messages from the retina to the brain.

Optic Nerve

The special nerve of the sense of sight which carries messages from the retina to the brain.

Optometrist

A licensed, non-medical practitioner, who measures reactive errors - that is, irregularities in the size or shape of the eyeball or surface of the cornea - and eye muscle disturbances. In his treatment the optometrist uses glasses, prisms and exercises only.

Ophthalmologist

A physician who specializes in refractive, medical, and surgical care of the eyes.

Optical device

Any system of lenses that enhances visual function.

Optotype

Letter, number, or symbol used in tests of visual abilities.

Orientation and mobility (O&M) instructor

A professional who specializes in teaching travel skills to persons with visual impairments.

P

Perimetry

Methods to determine an eye's filed of vision using objects that are moved from the nonseeing area to the seeing area or objects that are stationary but increased in intensity (static perimetry).

Photophobia

Abnormal sensitivity to and discomfort from light.

Posterior Chamber

Space between the back of the iris and the front of the lens; filled with aqueous fluid.

Presbyopia
A normal and gradual decrease in power of accommodation in the eye due to a physiological change that starts in middle age.

Prosthesis
An artificial substitute for a missing eye (or other missing part of the body).

Ptosis
A paralytic drooping of the upper lid.

Pupil
The round hole ("black" centre) in the middle of the iris which corresponds roughly with the lens opening of a camera; permits light to enter the eye.

R

Refractive Errors
A defect in the eye that prevents light rays from being brought to a single focus exactly on the retina; can be corrected with lenses.

Retina
Innermost lining of the eye, formed of sensitive nerve fibres (containing the light receptors - rods and cones) and connected with the optic nerve. (Converts the image into electrical signals which are transmitted along the optic nerve to the brain.)

Relative-distance magnification
Increasing the size of an image on the retina by increasing the size f an object to be viewed, such as large print.

Retina
The inner sensory nerve layer next to the choroid that lines the posterior two-thirds of the eyeball, which reacts to light and transmits impulses to the brain.

Retinitis pigmentosa
A group of progressive, often hereditary, retinal degenerative diseases characterized by decreasing peripheral vision; some cases progress to tunnel vision whereas others result in total blindness if the macula also becomes involved.

Retinal Detachment
A separation of the retina from the choroid which can lead to blindness.

Retinoblastoma
The most common malignant intraocular tumour of childhood - occurs usually under age five. It is probably always congenital (formerly known as glioma).

Retrolental Fibroplasia
A disease of the retina in which a mass of scar tissue forms at the back of the lens of the eye. Both eyes are affected in most cases, and it occurs chiefly in infants born prematurely who receive oxygen.

Rods
Cells of the retina mainly concerned with motion and vision at low degrees of illumination (night vision).

Rubella
German measles.

S
Saccadic eye movement
Rapid change in fixation from one point to another.

Scanning
The ability to search for a particular visual stimulus among other visual stimuli.

Sclera
The white part of the eye - a tough covering which, with the cornea, forms the external, protective coat of the eye.

Scotoma
A blind or partially blind area in the visual field.

Shifting gaze
Changing fixation to a new object of interest.

Snellen Chart
Used for testing central visual acuity. It consists of lines of letters, numbers or symbols in graded sizes drawn to Snellen measurements. Each side is labelled with the distance at which it cannot be read by the normal eye. Most often used for testing vision at a distance of 20 feet.

Spectacles
Eyeglasses that hold corrective lenses.

Strabismus
Squint; failure of the two eyes simultaneously to direct their gaze at the same object because of muscle imbalance.

Suspensory Ligament of the Lens
A delicate bundle -of fibres extending from the ciliary body to the lens for focusing at near or distant points.

T

Tangent screen perimetry
A flexible technique for examining visual fields with 30 degrees of fixation.

Teachers of students with visual impairments
A special trained and certified teacher who is qualified to teach special skills to students with visual impairments.

Telescope

A lens system that makes small objects appear closer and larger.

Trachoma

A form of infectious kerato-conjunctivitis caused by a specific virus which in the chronic form produces severe scarring of the eyelids and cornea.

Trauma

Injury, wound, shock or the resulting condition.

Tunnel Vision

(Gun barrel, tubular) Contraction of the visual field to such an extent that only a small area of central visual acuity remains, thus giving the affected individual the impression of looking through a tunnel.

Typoscope

Reading window or template made from card stock that allows a single word or line to be read.

V

Video magnifier

See Closed-circuit television system

Visually ability

Visually performance in real - world situations

Visual closure

Indentifying a form when only part of the form is presented.

Visual field

The entire region of space off to all sides that is visible when steadily looking and facing straight ahead.

Visual functions

Performance of the visual system in isolation and under standard measurement conditions; visual functions include visual acuity, visual fields, contrast sensitivity, color, response to light, oculomotor, control, accommodation, and so forth.

Visual impairment

Any degree of vision loss that cannot be corrected to normal through eyeglasses or contact lenses that affects an individual's ability to perform the tasks of daily life, caused by a visual system that is not working properly or not formed correctly.

Visually memory

The ability to remember a visual image or form after viewing.

Visual perception

The process of attaching meaning to a visual image.

Visual threshold

The smallest size of print that can be read at all at a given working distance.

Vision

The art or faculty of seeing; sight.

Visual Acuity

The sharpness or clearness of vision; the power of the eye to distinguish form as opposed to colour.

Vitreous Humour

Transparent, colourless mass of soft gelatinous material filling the eyeball behind the lens.

W

Working distance

The distance between the eye and an object or regard, such as a page being read.

References

Backman, 0. (1979) Low Vision Training, Liber, Hermods, Sweden.

Bailey, I.L and Lovie J.E (1976) New design principles for visual acuity letter charts", Am J Optom Physiol Opt, 53:740-745.

Baraga C (1980) Sequence of Visual Development, University of Texas, Austin.

Barraga, Natalie C, (1964) Increased Visual Behaviour in Low Vision Children. Research Series No. 13, American Foundation for the Blind, New York.

Barraga, Natalie C, (Ed.), (1980a) Program to Develop Efficiency in Visual Functioning source book on low vision. American Printing House for the Blind, Louisville.

Barraga., Natalie, C. (1970) Teachers Guide for Development of Visual Learning Abilities and Utilization of Low Vision. University of Texas, Austin.

Barraga., Natalie, C. (1976) Visual Handicaps and Learning a Developmental Approach. Wadsworth, California.

Barraga., Natalie, C. (1980b) Sequence of Visual Development. University of Texas, Austin.

Behrmann, P. (1975) Activities for Developing Visual Perception. Academic Therapy Publications, San Rafael.

Best, Tony, (1998) Assessment procedures for use with young visually handicapped children" (Part1). British **Journal of Visual Impairment** Autumn, Vol.5(3), P.85,87-88.

Brown, D., Simmons, V., & Methvin, J. (1991). The Oregon Project for Visually Impaired and Blind Preschool Children. Medford, Oregon: Jackson Education Service District.

Bush, W.J. & Giles, M.T. (1969) Aids to Psycholinguistic Teaching,.Charles E. Merrill, Columbia.

Chaman, E.K, Tobin M.J., Tooze F.H and Moss, S. (1979) Look and Think - A Handbook for 'Teachers, Royal National Institute for the Blind, London.

Chapman, E. (1979) Look and Think, a Handbook for Teachers, School Council Publication. London.

Chapman, Elizabeth K; Tobin, Michael J; Tooze, F H; Moss, S (1989), Look and think: a handbook for teachers, RNIB.

Corn, A. L. & Koenig, A.J. (1996) Foundations of Low Vision: Clinical and Functional Perspectives. New York: AFB Press.

Corn, A. L. & Koenig, A.J. (1996). Foundations of Low Vision: Clinical and Functional Perspectives. New York: AFB Press.

Corn, A. L., & Koenig, A.J. (1996) Foundations of Low vision. New York: American Foundation for the Blind.

Cratty, B.J and Sans, T.A. (1968) The Body Image, American Foundation for the Blind.

Cratty, B.J. (1971) Movement and Spatial Awareness in Blind Children and Youth, Charles C. Thomas, U.S.,

D'Andrea, F. M., & Farrenkopf, C. (2000) Looking to Learn: Promoting Literacy for Students with Low Vision. New York: AFB Press.

Davidson, Terry, A Survey on Developments in a New Field: Orientation and Mobility for the Low Vision Person, University of Pittsburgh, n.d.

Efron, M. & Duboff, B.R. (1976) A Vision Guide for Teachers of Deaf Blind Children, Raleigh, Division for Exceptional Children, North Carolina Dept. of Public Instruction.

Eleanor E Faye, M.D. (1984) Clinical Low Vision, 2nd edition, Little Brown and Company, Boston.

Ferrell, K. A. (1984) Parenting Preschoolers: Suggestions for Raising Young Blind and Visually Impaired Children. New York: American Foundation for the Blind.

Fraiberg., Selma, (1977) Insights from the Blind, Souvenir Press, London, 1977.

Friedman, Gerald R. (1976). Distance Low Vision Aids for Primary Level School Children. New Outlook for the Blind, Vol.70.

Gibson, E.J.(1969) Principles of Perceptual Learning and Development, Appleton-Century Crofts, New York.

Halliday., Carol, (1970) The Visually Impaired Child, Growth, Learning Development - Infancy to School Age, American Printing House for the Blind, Louisville.

Harrell, Lois J. (1977) Developmental Levels and Suggested Learning Activities, Clearinghouse Depository for Handicapped Students, California.

Hatlen, P. (1996) The Core Curriculum for Blind and Visually Impaired Students. Including those with Additional Disabilities. Review, 28(1), 25-32.

Hazecamp, J. & Huebner, M. (1989) Program Planning and Evaluation for Blind and Visually Impaired Students: National Guidelines for Educational Excellence. New York: AFB Press.

Hill, E. & Ponder, P. (1976) Orientation and Mobility Techniques, a Guide for the Practitioner, American Foundation for the Blind, New York.

Hyvarinen L.M.D. (1997) Identification and Assessment of Low Vision for Educational Purposes in Developing Countries, Part I, Addis Ababa.

Hyvärinen, L. (1988) Vision in Children, Normal and Abnormal. Canadian Deaf-Blind rubella Assoc, 41.

Hyvärinen, Lea **Lea Gratings (visual acuity test):** Small, Medium and Large Face Stimulus Paddle Precision Vision, Cat Nos: 2530, 2531, 2532.

Hyvärinen., Lea, (1997) Identification and Assessment of Low Vision for Educational Purposes in Developing Countries Part 1 Precision Vision, Finland.

Johns, J. L. (1997). Basic Reading Inventory: Pre-Primer through Grade Twelve & Early Literacy Assessments. Dubuque, Iowa: Kendall/Hunt Publishing Company.

Keeffe, J.E (1994) Assessment of Low Vision in Developing Countries Book 1. Screening for Impaired Vision, The University of Melbourne: World Health Organisation.

Keeffe, J.E (1994) Assessment of Low Vision in Developing Countries Book II. The Effects of Low Vision and Assessment of Functional Vision, The University of Melbourne: World Health Organisation.

Keeffe, J.E, Marie Crip, Mary O'Toole, Barbara Johnson and Louis Christi (1998) Visual Skill - A Curriculum Guide, Ministry of Education (Schools Division),

Victoria, Australia with the Common Wealth Education Department.

Keeffe, J.E. (1994) Assessment of Low Vision in Developing Countries Book 1. Screening for Impaired Vision, The University of Melbourne: World Health Organization

Keeffe, J.E. (1994). Assessment of Low Vision in Developing Countries Book II. The Effects of Low Vision and Assessment of Functional Vision, The University of Melbourne: World Health Organization

Koenig, A. J. & Holbrook, M. C. (1995) Learning Media Assessment of Students with Visual Impairments: A Resource Guide for Teachers 2nd Edition. Austin, Texas: Texas School for the Blind and Visually Impaired.

Koenig, A. J. & Holbrook, M.C. (1995) Learning Media Assessment of Students with Visual Impairments: A Resource Guide for Teachers 2nd Edition. Austin, Texas: Texas School for the Blind and Visually Impaired.

Koenig, A. J., & Holbrook, M. C. (Eds.) (2000). Foundations of Education, Vol. 2: Instructional Strategies for Teaching Children and Youths with Visual Impairments. New York: AFB Press.

Koenig, A. J., & Holbrook, M. C. (Eds.). (2000). Foundations of Education, Vol. 2: Instructional Strategies for Teaching Children and Youths with Visual Impairments. New York: AFB Press.

Levack, N. (1994) Low Vision: A Resource Guide with Adaptations for Students with Visual Impairments. Austin, Texas: Texas School for the Blind and Visually Impaired.

Levack, N. Annotated Bibliography of Curricular Materials Related to the Core Curriculum for Children and

Youths with Visual Impairments, Including Those with Multiple Disabilities. Austin, Texas: Texas School for the Blind and Visually Impaired.

Lovie- Kitchin., and Whittaker, D. (1993) Visual Requirements for Reading, Journal of Optometry Vision Sciences, Vol.70 (1), (54-65).

Lowenfeld, Berthold (Ed.), (1973) The Visually Handicapped Child in School, John Day, New York.

Lowenfeld, Berthold, (1981) On Blindness and Blind People, American Foundation for the Blind, New York.

Maplesden., Caroline, (1984) A Subjective Approach to Eccentric Viewing Training. Journal of Visual Impairment and Blindness, Vol. 78.

Montgomery County Public Schools, (1971) Vision Stimulation, Bulletin 227.

New Jersey Department of Education, Screening Children Ages 3 to 5.

O'Brien., Rosemary, (1976) Alive, Aware, a Person, Montgomery County Public Schools, Maryland,

Poggio, Gonzalez and Krause, (1998), Journal of Neuroscience, Vol 8, 4531-4550, Copyright © 1988 by Society for Neuroscience

Premavathy, V and Victoria, G (2006), Education of Children with Low Vision, RCI, Kanishka Publishers, New Delhi.

Psathas., George, (1976) Mobility, Orientation and Navigation Conceptual and Theoretical Considerations, New Outlook for the Blind, Vol.70.

Pugh, G. S., & Erin, J. (Eds.). (1999). Blind and Visually Impaired Students: Educational Service Guidelines. Watertown, MA: Perkins School for the Blind.

Quillman, RD., Low Vision Training Manual, College of Health and Human Services, Michigan, n.d.

Randall T Jose (1983) Understanding Low Vision, American Foundation for the Blind, New York.

Santhanaraj, V. (1999) Developing Visual Efficiency in Low Vision Children: See With the Blind, Books for Change, Bangalore& CBM, International, Germany, P.231-239.

Santhanaraj, V. (2000) A study of Children in India: Techniques and Materials to Increase Visual Effectiveness, Vision Rehabilitation: Assessment, Intervention and Outcomes, P.443-47.

Serras, F. & Nadler, R. (1981) One Step at a Time, New Jersey Commission for the Blind.

Sewell, D. (1997) Assessment Kit: Kit of Informal Tools for Academic Students with Visual Impairments. Austin, Texas: Texas School for the Blind and Visually Impaired.

Sheridan, Mary D. (1975) Children's Developmental Progress: the Stycar Sequences, NFE Publishing Co., Windsor.

Smith, A. & O'Donnell, M. (1992). Beyond Arms Reach. Philadelphia: Pennsylvania College of Optometry Press.

Swallow, R.M. et al (eds), (1978) A.F.B. Practice Report: Informal Assessment of Developmental Skills for Visually Handicapped Students, American Foundation for the Blind, New York.

Vijayan, P and Victoria, G, (2006), Education of Low Vision Children, Rehabilitation Council of India, Kanisha Publishers, New Delhi, India.

Vision Assessment and Prescription of Low Vision Devices (2004). Journal of Community Eye Health; 17(49): 3.

Warren, David H. (1977) Blindness and Early Childhood Development, American Foundation for the Blind, New York,

Webster, R. (1977) The Road to Freedom, a Parent Guide to Prepare the Blind Child to Travel Independently, Katon Publications, Jacksonville,

WHO-ICEVH (1992) Conference Report on Management of Low Vision in Children, Bangkok.

Wiener, Harold, (1977) Eyes OK, I'm OK, Academic Therapy Publications, California.

Wiener, W. & Vopata, A. (1980) Suggested Curriculum for Distance Vision Training with Optical Aids. Journal of Visual Impairment and Blindness, Vol.74.

World Health Organisation, (1997) Report on Global Initiative for the Elimination of Avoidable Blindness.

Online References

www.afb.org
www.afb.org
www.afb.org
www.afb.org/nationalagenda.asp
www.allaboutvision.com/eye-test
www.aph.org
www.aph.org
www.blind.msstate.edu/irr/def.html
www.boe.merc.k12.wv.us/osebps.htm#definition
www.brighthub.com/education/special/articles/35104.
aspx#ixzz18LS DtDCl
www.lighthouse.org
www.lowvisiononline.unimelb.edu.au/

www.suite101.com/content/
teaching-students-with-low-vision-a
www.suite101.com/content/teaching-students-with-low-
vision-a78264#ixzz18LQ y6NGn
www.ttc.gov/opa/2004/10/contactlens.shtm "The eye
chart and 20/20 vision"

Annexure
Functional Vision Assessment

Name   :
Standard :
School   :

Activities	Items given	Response

A. Visual Awareness
1. Respond to light
2. Aware of forms
3. Aware of 3D objects
4. Aware of 2D pictures
5. Aware of colours

B. Visual Attention
1. Attention to big object
2. Attention to small object
3. Attention at short distance
4. Attention at long distance
5. Attention to pictures

C. Visual Fixation
1. Fixation light at short distance
2. Fixation light at long distance

   3. Fixation object at short distance
   4. Fixation person at short distance
   5. Fixation person at long distance

D. Visual focusing
   1. Using both eyes to focus on object
   2. Using both eyes to focus on person
   3. Depth perception

E. Visual Tracking
   1. Tracking big object
   2. Tracking small object
   3. Tracking vertically
   4. Tracking horizontally
   5. Tracking circularly

F. Visual Scanning
   1. Scanning big object
   2. Scanning small object
   3. Scanning to identify details in object
   4. Scanning to identify details in picture
   5. Scanning in a surface

A. Visual Discrimination
   1. Discriminating 3D object
   2. Discriminating shapes
   3. Discriminating 2D objects
   4. Discriminating colours
   5. Discriminating textures

B. Visual Figure - Ground
   1. Identifying particular object in a group

2. Identifying particular object in a picture
3. Picking out a particular item in a group (pictures or objects)

C. Visual Memory
1. Recalling number of items seen in 1 minute
2. Recalling number of shapes in 1minute
3. Recalling the items in the picture
4. Recalling the clues in the known environment

D. Visual Closure
1. Identifying the whole object from the part
2. Identifying the missing details in picture
3. Identifying the missing letters

E. Spatial Relation and Form Constancy
1. Judging distance
2. Seeing object at different angles
3. Identifying objects at different positions

F. Visual Motor-Coordination
1. Moving in the known environment
2. Moving in the unknown environment
3. Performing hand-eye activities